Mediterranean Diet Guide Book

Choosing A Healthy Lifestyle

Darlene T. Grace

Contents

Chapter 1

Introduction

Food and culture are inextricably linked. We learn about delicious cuisine from our elders, who have learned the same thing from previous generations. As a result, public plans and preferences are developed and acquired, becoming an important part of our social identity that we carry with us regardless of where we live. A few families go so far as to have their own versions of the traditional foods, which are enviously cooked for all strangers. Societies are joining more than ever before, and varied cuisines are merging to create something completely unique and endemic, thanks to the wonders of modern mobility.

The Western countries are a fantastic example of public meals from all around the globe colliding in a single slow cooker. Seeing a row of national restaurants in the heart of a sophisticated city like Munich is no longer unusual, but the fact that one can order and eat actual kebabs and gyros at the same time is quite remarkable. Regardless of how varied they are, these numerous meals all have a common ancestor, one that can be traced back to the Mediterranean Sea region.

The Complete Mediterranean Diet 101

What is the Mediterranean Diet, and how does it differ from other eating plans?

The Mediterranean eating routine refers to the traditional eating habits and lifestyles of people living in the Mediterranean region, which includes Italy, Spain, France, Greece, and a few North African countries. The Mediterranean diet has recently gained a lot of popularity because people who live in these areas have better health and suffer from fewer diseases, such as cancer and cardiovascular disease. In this, food plays an important role.

This eating plan has numerous benefits, according to research. According to the findings of a recent study, eating the Mediterranean diet for a long time improved the cardiovascular health of many overweight and diabetic patients. In Spain, 7000 people participated in the survey. In this high-risk group, there was a 30% reduction in cardiovascular disease.

The New England Journal of Medicine published the findings, which shocked the world. Several studies have shown that the Mediterranean diet can help to balance blood sugar, prevent Alzheimer's disease, lower the risk of heart disease and stroke, improve brain health, reduce anxiety and depression, aid weight loss, and even lower the risk of certain cancers.

Because of social, ethnic, agrarian, strict, and monetary differences, eating habits differ from country to country and even within these countries' locales. As a result, there is no such thing as a typical Mediterranean diet. There are a few common factors in any case.

Diet Pyramid of the Mediterranean

The Mediterranean diet food pyramid is a nutrition guide that teaches people how to eat the right foods in the right amounts and at the right times, as dictated by traditional Mediterranean eating habits.

The World Health Organization, Harvard School of Public Health, and the Prior Ways Preservation Trust collaborated to create the pyramid in 1993.

The pyramid has six food layers, with active work at the bottom, which is an important part of maintaining a healthy lifestyle.

The main food layer, which includes whole grains, breads, beans, pasta, and nuts, is located just above it. It's the deepest layer, with food options that follow the Mediterranean diet's guidelines. Then there are the greens. As you progress up the pyramid, you'll notice food sources that should be consumed less frequently, with the highest layer containing food varieties that should be avoided or limited.

The food pyramid for the Mediterranean diet is easy to understand. It explains how to stick to the eating plan in a straightforward way.

Layers in Food

Whole Grains, Breads, and Beans - The shortest and longest layer, with food sources that are unmistakably recommended. For the most part, these ingredients should be used in your meals. Eat whole wheat bread, pita, whole wheat rolls and buns, whole grain oats, whole wheat pasta, and earthy colored rice. You can get a lot of nutrition by eating 4 to 6 servings a day.

Fruits and vegetables are almost as important as the layer that has been reduced. A variety of non-bland vegetables, such as asparagus, broccoli, beets, tomatoes, carrots, cucumber, cabbage, cauliflower, and turnips, should be consumed on a daily basis. Day by day, 4–8 servings 2–4 servings of natural products should be consumed on a regular basis. New fruits should be picked on occasion.

Extra-virgin olive oil should be used to cook your suppers. Daily use It is beneficial to the body because it lowers the levels of low-density lipoprotein (LDL) and total cholesterol. Olive oil may be used up to 2 tablespoons. Canola oil is also permitted in the eating regimen. Fish - We've arrived at the food layers, which must be consumed weekly rather than daily. Fish can be consumed two to three times per week. Fish, herring, salmon, and sardines are excellent greasy ocean fish. Ocean fish contain heart-healthy omega-3 unsaturated fats as well as a high protein content. Mussels, shellfish, shrimp, and mollusks are all excellent shellfish options.

Poultry, cheddar, and yogurt - Cheese, yogurt, eggs, chicken, and other poultry products should all be included in the diet, but only in moderation. During the course of seven days, you will experience the most extreme conditions 2-3 times. Dairy products that are low in fat are best. It is preferable to use soy milk, cheddar cheese, or yogurt.

Meats and desserts are the highest layer of food sources to avoid. You are only allowed to have them once a month. Keep in mind that the Mediterranean is one of the most beautiful regions on the planet.

Plant-based meals are part of my daily routine. Meat, especially red meat, has almost no place to be found. Take red meat in small amounts if you can't live without it. Choose cuts that are leaner. Just to celebrate, have desserts. After following the eating plan for a month, you can indulge in two or three desserts.

Foods to Consume

Many residents of the district, for example, consume a diet rich in whole grains, vegetables, natural products, nuts, seeds, fish, fats, and vegetables. It isn't as restrictive as some low-fat diets. Indeed, fat is beneficial, but only when consumed in moderation, such as polyunsaturated fat (omega-3 unsaturated fats) found in fish and monounsaturated fat found in olive oil.

It's completely plant-based, but it's also not vegan. The eating plan recommends limiting your intake of saturated and trans fats, which can be found in red meat and other processed foods. You should likewise restrict the admission of dairy products.

Fruits and vegetables – Eat daily. Try to have 7-10 servings every day. Meals are strongly based on plant-based foods. Eat fresh fruits and vegetables. Pick from seasonal varieties.

Whole grains – Eat whole-grain cereal, bread, and pasta. All parts of whole grains – the germ, bran, and the endosperm provide healthy nutrients. These nutrients are lost when the grain is refined into white flour.

Healthy fats only – Avoid butter for cooking. Switch to olive oil. Dip your bread in flavored olive oil instead of applying margarine or butter on bread. Trans fats and saturated fats can cause heart disease.

Fish – Fish is encouraged. Eat fatty fish like herring, mackerel, albacore tuna, sardines, lake trout, and salmon. Fatty fish will give you plenty of healthy omega-3 fatty acids that reduce inflammations. Omega-3 fatty acids also reduced blood clotting, decreased triglycerides, and improves heart health. Eat fresh seafood two times

a week. Avoid deep-fried fish. Choose grilled fish.

Legumes – Provides the body with minerals, protein, complex carbohydrates, polyunsaturated fatty acids, and fiber. Eat daily.

Dairy and poultry – You can eat eggs, milk products, and chicken throughout the week, but with moderation. Restrict cheese. Go for plain or low-fat Greek yogurt instead of cheese.

Nuts and seeds – 3 or more servings every week. Eat a variety of nuts, seeds, and beans. Walnuts and almonds are all allowed.

Red meat – The Mediterranean diet is not meat-based. You can still have red meat, but only once or twice a week max. If you love red meat, then make sure that it is lean. Take small portions only. Avoid processed meats like salami, sausage, and bologna.

Olive Oil – The key source of fat. Olive oil will give you monounsaturated fat that lowers the LDL or low-density lipoprotein cholesterol and total cholesterol level. Seeds and nuts will also provide you monounsaturated fat. You can also have canola oil but no cream, butter, mayonnaise, or margarine. Take up to 4 tablespoons of olive oil a day. For best results, only take extra-virgin olive oil.

Wine – Red wine is allowed, but with moderation. Don't take more than a glass of red wine daily. Best take only 3-4 days a week.

Desserts – Say no to ice cream, sweets, pies, and chocolate cake. Fresh fruits are good.

Main Components– Focus on natural foods – Avoid processed foods as much as you can

Be flexible – Plan to have a variety of foods

Consume fruits, vegetables, healthy fats, and whole grains daily Have weekly plans for poultry, fish, eggs, and beans

Take dairy products moderately

Limit red meat intake

Take water instead of soda. Only take wine when you are having a meal.

Foods in the Traditional Mediterranean Diet Whole Vegetables Grains

Chapter 2

Brown Artichokes

rice Oats Arugula Bulgur Beats Fruits Protein Dairy Others Apples Almonds Apricots Avocados Walnuts Pistachios Barley Broccoli Figs

Farrow Cucumbers Wheat Eggplant berries Pasta Onions Whole Spinach grain bread Olives

Strawberries

Tomatoes Melons

Cannellini Beans Chickpeas Kidney beans

Salmon Tuna

Low/non-fat plain Bay or Greek yogurt leaf Manchego cheese Basil Brie cheese Olive oil Ricotta cheese Red wine Parmesan cheese Mint Feta cheese Pepper cumin Garlic Couscous Potatoes Grapes Eggs Anise spice

Foods Allowed

You ought to eat a lot of organic products, vegetables, nuts, seeds, beans, entire grains, spices, and vegetables. Olive oil and canola oil are both allowed.

Eat Moderately

Fish, fish, chicken, eggs, low-fat cheddar, and yogurt.

Restricted Foods

This rundown incorporates refined grains like white rice, white bread, desserts, prepared items, and pop. Likewise, confine handled meats and red meat. Keep an eye out for high-fat dairy items like spread and frozen yogurt and trans-fats in margarine and handled foods.

Med Diet Serving Sizes

Food Groups and Serving Sizes (Daily/Weekly)

4–8 servings of non-starchy vegetables

2–4 servings of fruits

12 cup cooked vegetables or 1 cup raw vegetables per serving

Asparagus, artichokes, broccoli, beets, Brussels sprouts, cabbage, celery, cauliflower, carrots, eggplant, tomatoes, cucumber, onion, zucchini, turnips, mushrooms, and salad greens are some of the vegetables that can be used.

Potatoes, peas, and corn are all starchy vegetables. A small fruit, 12 cup juice, or 14 cup dried fruit counts as one serving.

Fruits are high in nutrients and fiber, so eat them. You can also eat canned fruits with their juice and frozen fruits that haven't been sweetened.

Nuts, legumes, and seeds

4 servings of seeds

2 to 3 servings of low-fat dairy

12 cup cooked kidney, pinto, garbanzo, soy, navy beans, lentils, or split peas, or 14 cup fat-free beans equals one serving of legumes.

2 tablespoons sesame or sunflower seeds, 1 tablespoon peanut butter, 7-8 pecans or walnuts, 12-15 almonds, 20 peanuts = 1 serving of nuts and seeds. 1-2 servings of nuts or seeds and 1-2 servings of legumes are recommended. Whole nuts provide unsaturated fat without raising LDL cholesterol levels, while legumes provide minerals, fiber, and protein.

1 cup skim milk, nonfat yogurt, or 1 oz. low-fat cheese per serving

Soy yogurt, calcium-rich soy milk, or soy cheese can be used in place of dairy products. If you eat less than 2 servings per day, you should take a vitamin D and calcium supplement.

Fish – up to three times per week

1 to 3 times per week, poultry

4 to 6 servings of whole grains and starchy vegetables

4 to 6 servings of healthy fats

3 ounces equals one serving

Cooking methods include baking, sautéing, roasting, broiling, poaching, and grilling. Fatty fish, such as sardines, herring, salmon, or mackerel, are best. Fish is high in omega-3 fats, which have numerous health benefits. 3 ounces equals one serving

The poultry can be sautéed, baked, grilled, or stir-fried. Remove the skin before eating. 1 ounce of– is one serving.

12 CUP SUGAR POTATOES, POTATOES, POTATOES, POTATOES, POTATOES, POTATOES, P 1 whole-wheat bread slice

1 whole-grain roll, small

6 whole-grain crackers 12 large whole-grain bun Pita bread (whole wheat, 6-inch diameter)

12 cup brown rice, whole-wheat pasta, or barley, cooked 12 cup cereal (whole grains) (cracked wheat, oatmeal, quinoa)

Whole grains are high in fiber and help to keep the stomach full, which aids in weight loss. a serving of –

1 tablespoon salad dressing (regular) 2 tablespoons salad dressing (light) 2 tblsp margarine (light)

1 tsp. olive or canola oil 1 teaspoon mayonnaise (regular) a quarter of an avocado olives (five)

Because these fats are mostly unsaturated, your LDL cholesterol levels will not rise.

Men should limit themselves to two drinks per day. Women should limit themselves to one drink per day. A maximum of one drink per day is permitted. alcoholic beverage ounces (vodka, whiskey, brandy, etc.). If you have high triglycerides or blood pressure, stay away from alcohol.

The Mediterranean Way of Life

Not only is food important, but so is living a healthy lifestyle. This includes getting enough exercise as well as making social connections.

Physical activity is at the bottom of the food pyramid, even below the first and most important food layer - getting enough actual work is essential. This includes regular practice, swimming, hiking, running, and playing a functional game. In any case, there are other options for maintaining good health.

Many people from the Mediterranean region do not go to the recreation center. They are not, however, idle. Many people are engaged in a great deal of difficult work. They'll take a stroll to their workplace, the pastry kitchen, or the farmer's market. They take a stroll to their friend's house. Even a daily walk and some moderate exercise can be beneficial. It's fantastic to see consistent progress. Keep your distance from the elevator. Instead, take the stairwell.

How much practice is sufficient? Working out is beneficial to one's health 100 percent of the time. You do not, however, need to lift any loads. 5 days a week, 10-15 minutes on the treadmill and rec center bicycle should suffice. 30 minutes of moderate-intensity exercise will suffice. Not much if you can do a couple of muscle-reinforcing exercises twice a day seven days a week. You could also try walking for 200 minutes five times a week or gardening for an hour four times a week.

Cook at Home - Eating at home is always preferable to eating out. Café cooked pasta, for example, will have a higher sodium content. Instead of the heavy cream sauce, you can have one part whole grain spaghetti with pureed tomatoes and spinach. Setting up the suppers at home allows you to take care of the fixings. Home-cooked meals are high in minerals, nutrients, and fiber, as well as low in added sugar, sodium, and saturated fat.

Eat with others - Dinner should be a social occasion. Eating with friends or family is a fantastic way to relieve stress. It will improve your mood, which will have a significant impact on your overall health. Furthermore, it will prevent you from overeating. You'll see the Mediterranean public eating together in a garden on a regular basis.

Turn off the television and enjoy your meal. Keep an eye on what the kids are eating. If you live alone, invite a colleague, neighbor, or companion over. You could invite someone over and plan dinners together.

Laugh Often - Have you heard the old adage, "Laughter is the best pain reliever there is"? In Mediterranean culture, this is true. There are a lot of people who have a lot of personality.

Their conversations are full of wit. They enjoy telling stories. Appreciate life and maintain a positive outlook/

Consider food as an example of living a simple life. You won 't observe them purchasing a lot of anything. They've never bought anything in bulk before. They purchase crisp, zeroing in on every day needs. Also obviously, new food is generally best. Enjoy Every Bite - Slow down and partake in each chomp. Many will eat for endurance. However, in the Mediterranean belt, they love their food. They appreciate it. Try not to eat in a hurry. Plunk down and have an appropriate meal.

Health Benefits of the Med Diet

Heart illness and stroke - The Mediterranean eating routine suggests restricted eating of handled food sources, red meat, and refined breads, which contributes towards a lower hazard of heart sicknesses and stroke. A review did more than 12 years among 25,000 ladies observed that ladies eating this diet had the option to decrease their gamble of coronary illness by 25 percent .

The PREDIMED (1) study was completed among men and women with a high-hazard of cardiovascular sickness and type-2 diabetes in Spain. Following 5 years of exploration, it was found that the people who had a calorie-unhindered Mediterranean eating regimen had a 30 percent lower hazard of heart issues.

Alzheimer's - Research additionally recommends that the eating routine can further develop glucose levels, cholesterol, and vein wellbeing, which thusly may bring down the gamble of dementia and Alzheimer's sickness. A recent report (2) filtered the minds of 70 individuals for dementia and observed their food propensities. Following 2 years, it was seen that those on the Mediterranean eating routine had less protein plaques or beta-amyloid stores than others, and in this manner a lower hazard of Alzheimer's.

Other investigations have likewise uncovered that the Mediterranean eating regimen may likewise forestall the decay of reasoning abilities and memory with age as there is an expanded stock of oxygen and supplements to the brain.

The eating regimen is loaded with cancer prevention agents, for example, olive oil and nuts, which might postpone cognitive deterioration. A connection between consuming fish and lower hazard of Alzheimer's has likewise been found.

Diabetes - The eating routine with sound carbs and entire grains offers large advantages like balancing out the glucose level. Wheat berries, buckwheat, and quinoa are examples of complex whole grain carbohydrates that boost overall energy and keep blood sugar levels stable. The Mediterranean dietary pattern has been shown to reduce the risk of type-2 diabetes by 52 percent in over 400 people aged 55 to 80. This research took almost 4 years to complete.

Parkinson's disease - The diet is high in cell reinforcements, which may reduce the risk of Parkinson's disease by as much as 50 percent by preventing oxidative stress or cell damage.

Weight gain - The Mediterranean diet is high in fiber, which makes you feel full. You won't be able to eat as much. The eating plan improves digestion while also promoting weight loss. Instead of simple carbohydrates, focus on stringy veggies, organic goods, legumes, and vegetables. Because almost nothing is forbidden in the general feast diet, it is a safe and sustainable approach of becoming more fit. Mediterranean eating habits were ranked first in the 'Best Overall Diet' category by U.S. News & World Report in 2019. Cancer - A healthy diet has also been linked to a reduced risk of some types of cancer. Analysts analyzed the findings of 83 studies involving millions of people and hypothesized that it might reduce the risk of breast, gastric, colorectal, and colon cancer. Individuals who follow this dietary plan have a much decreased incidence of malignant growth mortality. The increased acceptance of whole grains, veggies, and organic goods has been attributed to this. This study's findings were published in the journal Nutrients.

According to another study published in the JAMA Internal Medicine journal, women who followed this diet had a 62 percent lower risk of developing breast cancer.

Inflammation - Omega-3 unsaturated fats found in fatty fish such as fish, mackerel, and salmon may help to reduce inflammation. Omega-3 will also improve your skin's flexibility and strength.

Rheumatoid arthritis - In this immune system illness, the body's invulnerable framework unintentionally attacks the joints, creating swelling and pain. Long-chain omega-3 unsaturated fats, such as those found in oily fish, have been suggested by the National Institutes of Health's Office of Dietary Supplements to aid with the symptoms of RA.

Because it is a plant-based eating plan with a ton of natural products, veggies, nuts, seeds, and vegetables, the Med diet delivers 7 percent more good bacteria in the microbiome than those on a traditional western eating regimen. The health of the stomach is improved even more as a result of this.

What You Should Do First

The most straightforward way to start an eating routine is to make little changes. Gradually incorporate more of the Mediterranean diet's recommended foods while avoiding those that aren't.

To begin, keep butter to a minimum. Use olive oil instead of butter to sauté your food.

At every meal, include fresh fruits and vegetables. For dessert, eat fruits. Replace red meat with fish. Sea fish with a lot of fat is a good choice.

Breads, pastas, and rice that have been refined should be avoided. Complete grains should be consumed.

High-fat dairy products should be avoided. Only a small amount of cheese should be used.

Once a week, try to eat vegetarian or vegan. As you get more into the diet, make this twice a week. Vegetables, whole grains, and beans should all be a part of your diet. To make it more interesting, use spices and herbs.

Breakfast is a must.Food Groups and Serving Sizes (Daily/Weekly)

4–8 servings of non-starchy vegetables

2–4 servings of fruits

12 cup cooked vegetables or 1 cup raw vegetables per serving

Asparagus, artichokes, broccoli, beets, Brussels sprouts, cabbage, celery, cauliflower, carrots, eggplant, tomatoes, cucumber, onion, zucchini, turnips, mushrooms, and salad greens are some of the vegetables that can be used.

Potatoes, peas, and corn are all starchy vegetables. A small fruit, 12 cup juice, or 14 cup dried fruit counts as one serving.

Fruits are high in nutrients and fiber, so eat them. You can also eat canned fruits with their juice and frozen fruits that haven't been sweetened.

Nuts, legumes, and seeds

4 servings of seeds

2 to 3 servings of low-fat dairy

12 cup cooked kidney, pinto, garbanzo, soy, navy beans, lentils, or split peas, or 14 cup fat-free beans equals one serving of legumes.

2 tablespoons sesame or sunflower seeds, 1 tablespoon peanut butter, 7-8 pecans or walnuts, 12-15 almonds, 20 peanuts = 1 serving of nuts and seeds. 1-2 servings of nuts or seeds and 1-2 servings of legumes are recommended. Whole nuts provide unsaturated fat without raising LDL cholesterol levels, while legumes provide minerals, fiber, and protein.

1 cup skim milk, nonfat yogurt, or 1 oz. low-fat cheese per serving

Soy yogurt, calcium-rich soy milk, or soy cheese can be used in place of dairy products. If you eat less than 2 servings per day, you should take a vitamin D and calcium supplement.

Fish – up to three times per week

1 to 3 times per week, poultry

4 to 6 servings of whole grains and starchy vegetables

4 to 6 servings of healthy fats

3 ounces equals one serving

Cooking methods include baking, sautéing, roasting, broiling, poaching, and grilling. Fatty fish, such as sardines, herring, salmon, or mackerel, are best. Fish is high in omega-3 fats, which have numerous health benefits. 3 ounces equals one serving

The poultry can be sautéed, baked, grilled, or stir-fried. Remove the skin before eating. 1 ounce of– is one serving.

12 CUP SUGAR POTATOES, POTATOES, POTATOES, POTATOES, POTATOES, POTATOES, P 1 whole-wheat bread slice

1 whole-grain roll, small

6 whole-grain crackers 12 large whole-grain bun Pita bread (whole wheat, 6-inch diameter)

12 cup brown rice, whole-wheat pasta, or barley, cooked 12 cup cereal (whole grains) (cracked wheat, oatmeal, quinoa)

Whole grains are high in fiber and help to keep the stomach full, which aids in weight loss. a serving of –

1 tablespoon salad dressing (regular) 2 tablespoons salad dressing (light) 2 tblsp margarine (light)

1 tsp. olive or canola oil 1 teaspoon mayonnaise (regular) a quarter of an avocado olives (five)

Because these fats are mostly unsaturated, your LDL cholesterol levels will not rise.

Men should limit themselves to two drinks per day. Women should limit themselves to one drink per day. A maximum of one drink per day is permitted. alcoholic beverage ounces (vodka, whiskey, brandy, etc.). If you have high triglycerides or blood pressure, stay away from alcohol.

The Mediterranean Way of Life

Not only is food important, but so is living a healthy lifestyle. This includes getting enough exercise as well as making social connections.

Physical activity is at the bottom of the food pyramid, even below the first and most important food layer - getting enough actual work is essential. This includes regular practice, swimming, hiking, running, and playing a functional game. In any case, there are other options for maintaining good health.

Many people from the Mediterranean region do not go to the recreation center. They are not, however, idle. Many people are engaged in a great deal of difficult work. They'll take a stroll to their workplace, the pastry kitchen, or the farmer's market. They take a stroll to their friend's house. Even a daily walk and some moderate exercise can be beneficial. It's fantastic to see consistent progress. Keep your distance from the elevator. Instead, take the stairwell.

How much practice is sufficient? Working out is beneficial to one's health 100 percent of the time. You do not, however, need to lift any loads. 5 days a week, 10-15 minutes on the treadmill and rec center bicycle should suffice. 30 minutes of moderate-intensity exercise will suffice. Not much if you can do a couple of muscle-reinforcing exercises twice a day seven days a week. You could also try walking for 200 minutes five times a week or gardening for an hour four times a week.

Cook at Home - Eating at home is always preferable to eating out. Café cooked pasta, for example, will have a higher sodium content. Instead of the heavy cream sauce, you can have one part whole grain spaghetti with pureed tomatoes and spinach. Setting up the suppers at home allows you to take care of the fixings. Home-cooked meals are high in minerals, nutrients, and fiber, as well as low in added sugar, sodium, and saturated fat.

Eat with others - Dinner should be a social occasion. Eating with friends or family is a fantastic way to relieve stress. It will improve your mood, which will have a significant impact on your overall health. Furthermore, it will prevent you from overeating. You'll see the Mediterranean public eating together in a garden on a regular basis.

Turn off the television and enjoy your meal. Keep an eye on what the kids are eating. If you live alone, invite a colleague, neighbor, or companion over. You could invite someone over and plan dinners together.

Laugh Often - Have you heard the old adage, "Laughter is the best pain reliever there is"? In Mediterranean culture, this is true. There are a lot of people who have a lot of personality.

Their conversations are full of wit. They enjoy telling stories. Appreciate life and maintain a positive outlook/

Consider food as an example of living a simple life. You won't observe them purchasing a lot of anything. They've never bought anything in bulk before. They purchase crisp, zeroing in on every day needs. Also obviously, new food is generally best. Enjoy Every Bite - Slow down and partake in each chomp. Many will eat for endurance. However, in the Mediterranean belt, they love their food. They appreciate it. Try not to eat in a hurry. Plunk down and have an appropriate meal.

Health Benefits of the Med Diet

Heart illness and stroke - The Mediterranean eating routine suggests restricted eating of handled food sources, red meat, and refined breads, which contributes towards a lower hazard of heart sicknesses and stroke. A review did more than 12 years among 25,000 ladies observed that ladies eating this diet had the option to decrease their gamble of coronary illness by 25 percent .

The PREDIMED (1) study was completed among men and women with a high-hazard of cardiovascular sickness and type-2 diabetes in Spain. Following 5 years of exploration, it was found that the people who had a calorie-unhindered Mediterranean eating regimen had a 30 percent lower hazard of heart issues.

Alzheimer's - Research additionally recommends that the eating routine can further develop glucose levels, cholesterol, and vein wellbeing, which thusly may bring down the gamble of dementia and Alzheimer's sickness. A recent report (2) filtered the minds of 70 individuals for dementia and observed their food propensities. Following 2 years, it was seen that those on the Mediterranean eating routine had less protein plaques or beta-amyloid stores than others, and in this manner a lower hazard of Alzheimer's.

Other investigations have likewise uncovered that the Mediterranean eating regimen may likewise forestall the decay of reasoning abilities and memory with age as there is an expanded stock of oxygen and supplements to the brain.

The eating regimen is loaded with cancer prevention agents, for example, olive oil and nuts, which might postpone cognitive deterioration. A connection between consuming fish and lower hazard of Alzheimer's has likewise been found.

Diabetes - The eating routine with sound carbs and entire grains offers large advantages like balancing out the glucose level. Wheat berries, buckwheat, and quinoa are examples of complex whole grain carbohydrates that boost overall energy and keep blood sugar levels stable. The Mediterranean dietary pattern has been shown to reduce the risk of type-2 diabetes by 52 percent in over 400 people aged 55 to 80. This research took almost 4 years to complete.

Parkinson's disease - The diet is high in cell reinforcements, which may reduce the risk of Parkinson's disease by as much as 50 percent by preventing oxidative stress or cell damage.

Weight gain - The Mediterranean diet is high in fiber, which makes you feel full. You won't be able to eat as much. The eating plan improves digestion while also promoting weight loss. Instead of simple carbohydrates, focus on stringy veggies, organic goods, legumes, and vegetables. Because almost nothing is forbidden in the general feast diet, it is a safe and sustainable approach of becoming more fit. Mediterranean eating habits were ranked first in the 'Best Overall Diet' category by U.S. News & World Report in 2019. Cancer - A healthy diet has also been linked to a reduced risk of some types of cancer. Analysts analyzed the findings of 83 studies involving millions of people and hypothesized that it might reduce the risk of breast, gastric, colorectal, and colon cancer. Individuals who follow this dietary plan have a much decreased incidence of malignant growth mortality. The increased acceptance of whole grains, veggies, and organic goods has been attributed to this. This study's findings were published in the journal Nutrients.

According to another study published in the JAMA Internal Medicine journal, women who followed this diet had a 62 percent lower risk of developing breast cancer.

Inflammation - Omega-3 unsaturated fats found in fatty fish such as fish, mackerel, and salmon may help to reduce inflammation. Omega-3 will also improve your skin's flexibility and strength.

Rheumatoid arthritis - In this immune system illness, the body's invulnerable framework unintentionally attacks the joints, creating swelling and pain. Long-chain omega-3 unsaturated fats, such as those found in oily fish, have been suggested by the National Institutes of Health's Office of Dietary Supplements to aid with the symptoms of RA.

Because it is a plant-based eating plan with a ton of natural products, veggies, nuts, seeds, and vegetables, the Med diet delivers 7 percent more good bacteria in the microbiome than those on a traditional western eating regimen. The health of the stomach is improved even more as a result of this.

What You Should Do First

The most straightforward way to start an eating routine is to make little changes. Gradually incorporate more of the Mediterranean diet's recommended foods while avoiding those that aren't.

To begin, keep butter to a minimum. Use olive oil instead of butter to sauté your food.

At every meal, include fresh fruits and vegetables. For dessert, eat fruits. Replace red meat with fish. Sea fish with a lot of fat is a good choice.

Breads, pastas, and rice that have been refined should be avoided. Complete grains should be consumed.

High-fat dairy products should be avoided. Only a small amount of cheese should be used.

Once a week, try to eat vegetarian or vegan. As you get more into the diet, make this twice a week. Vegetables, whole grains, and beans should all be a part of your diet. To make it more interesting, use spices and herbs.

Breakfast is a must.

When rushing to work, a lot of people forget to eat breakfast. This is never a good idea because your body will assume there isn't enough food and slow down digestion, potentially leading to weight gain.

English biscuits, whole grain toast, hummus-filled bagels, delicate cheddar, nut margarine, or avocado are all good options. A cup of berries or a medium-sized natural product should be added. You'll stay fuller longer thanks to the fiber. A few nuts and an egg can also be included. A few times a month, bacon or a hotdog are permitted. A bowl of soup, for example, will be of great assistance.

Dessert

In the Mediterranean diet, the treat you should eat isn't the same as what you'd eat on a regular basis in the United States. Desserts and frozen yogurt, for example, are strictly prohibited. Cakes, treats, and cakes should also be avoided or limited. You can probably eat them once or twice a month.

For dessert, opt for organic options. If you get tired of something, you can be inventive.

Using organic goods on a regular basis. You might, for example, grill pineapple and drizzle honey on top. Fill a date or fig with goat cheese. Add a few nuts to the mix. Poach your pear in some honey and pomegranate juice. You may also make a whole wheat natural product tar. There are so many different ways to spice up your sweet.

After dinner, several Mediterranean civilizations will enjoy a glass of red wine. Although research has shown that consuming red wine offers health benefits, not everyone is convinced. If you've never had wine before, don't start now.

Top 7 Mediterranean Diet Lifestyle Success Tips

Make a plan for your suppers - Make a list of what you'll eat for supper and when you'll eat it. Plan what you'll eat when you have the chance and the willpower at the conclusion of the week. This also applies to the snacks. Then double-check that you have all of the essential materials on hand ahead of time. Over time, it will get easier for you to consume sound. You may prepare a few suppers ahead of time, especially ones that can be refrigerated.

Use olive oil instead of coconut or vegetable oil for cooking. The use of extra-virgin olive oil is strongly recommended. Olive oil contains monounsaturated unsaturated fats, which help to raise HDL cholesterol levels (the great sort). According to a recent study, HDL cholesterol may even remove LDL particles from the corridors. To enhance the taste of your dish, drizzle it with olive oil.

Days without meat - The Mediterranean diet is mostly plant-based, with some fish. You can get all of the proteins you need from heartbeats, beans, and seafood. Meat is only allowed to be consumed on more than one occasion every month. Red meat is inferior than chicken.

Adopt - Mediterranean tastes aren't always compatible with all culinary techniques. In any case, you may take on a variety of components. You may use oils containing unsaturated fats, for example, while preparing a spicy dish like curry. Olive oil is fantastic. Palm and coconut oil are inferior than sunflower and rapeseed oil.

Antioxidants - Consume antioxidant-rich veggies and organic goods. You'll get pterostilbene, resveratrol, and glutathione from this. Onions, garlic, cruciferous vegetables, and spinach are all good sources of glutathione. Resveratrol may be found in raspberries and blueberries. Other vital cell reinforcements for superb health are oregano, mint, basil, and other spices.

Eat healthy - Pasta, a popular Italian dish from the Mediterranean, is also included in the plan. Focus on whole grain options, but you'll discover that if you don't have any, you'll end up with more grains.

Snacking As a snack, have nuts. Carry a small bag of cashews, pistachios, or almonds with you at all times. They're all highly satisfying in their own right. The Nutrition Journal published a study that found that those who substituted almonds for chips, sweets, cereal bars, and wafers consumed less empty calories, salt, and added sugar. Nuts will also provide you with essential nutrients and fiber.

Breakfast Meal Plan for a Week

Frittata with rainbow colors 1 serving grilled tomatoes, whole-wheat bread, and 1 fried egg

Dijon Salmon with GreenGreen salad with Bean Pilaf – 1 serving, or hummus and pita bed– whole-grain pizza with 1 serve, or 2 cups of green veggies and salad greens with olives tomato sauce To increase the number of calories in ham or chicken, add tuna and cherry tomatoes.

Breakfast, Lunch, and Dinner on Day 2

Linguine with mushroom salad and Brussels sprouts 1 serving muesli with chickpeas or raspberries 1 cup Greek yogurt (1 serve)

12 sauce– 1 serving, or a whole-grain sandwich with salmon or baked cod 1portion zucchini with black pepper eggplant, onion, bell pepper, and garlic for taste. You

a cup of blueberries or a pinch of pepper Avocado or nectarines, diced, should be spread on top. For added calories, spread hummus on your toast.

On day 3, add 1 baked potato with chives to your meal. Ricotta and fig toast for breakfast, lunch, or dinner, or 1 cup whole grain oats with dates, honey, and cinnamon. 1 oz. crushed almonds are also a good addition.

Spiced boiled beans with garlic, cumin, and laurel. Arugula salad with cucumber, feta cheese, tomato, and olive oil dressing is also available.

1 serving of quinoa or tomato-sauced cod Half cup whole-grain spaghetti with olive oil, grilled veggies, and tomato sauce is another option. Breakfast and Lunch on Day 4

1 dish creamed pecan and blueberry oats, or 2 scrambled eggs with onions, tomatoes, and bell peppers

A plate of Brussels sprouts salad or roasted anchovies on whole-grain bread with lemon juice is a delicious option. 2 cups kale and 2 cups steamed tomatoes

Dinner

1 cup spinach with herbs and lemon juice, or 1 serve quinoa chickpea bowl Combine the boiled artichoke, salt, garlic powder, and olive oil in a mixing bowl. Day 5: Breakfast, Lunch, and Dinner Garlic Chicken Pasta

2 cups steaming kale with cucumber, tomato, and lemon juice or stuffed olive fish with oregano and lemon

Raspberries in Muesli 1 cup Greek tomatoes, red pepper, basil, honey-infused yogurt, baby spinach, and Italian cinnamon Add a pinch of salt and pepper, or a cup of quinoa with tomatoes and an apple if desired. bell peppers, and olives Olives and parmesan cheese Breakfast, Lunch, and Dinner on Day 6 Broccoli and shrimp in a skillet with mild cheese Cobb salad with parsley, oregano, garlic, onion, omelet with Romanocucumber, yogurt, baby olive oil, tomatoes, cheese, broccoli florets, spinach, eggs, avocado, parsley, shrimp, and 2 percent milk, parsley, tomatoes, bacon strips, and feta cheese, or oveneggs, or 2 slices of whole feta cheese, or 1 cup of feta cheese

Grain toast topped with soft mixed greens, queso fresco, cucumber, and tomato.

or ricotta cheese

Carrots, artichokes, eggplant, zucchini, tomato, and sweet potatoes can all be roasted.

Brunch and Lunch Tomato bites with basil, oregano from Mediterranean chickpeas, Gouda cheese, garlic, onion, and olive oil

Dinner 1 serving Mediterranean chicken with olives or yogurt and honey fruit cups with orange zest, almonds, and fruits such as bananas, grapes, apples, and pears

or 2 cups oil, artichoke, oregano, and orzo

stewed arugula with olives, olive zucchini, onion, potato, oil, and tomato, or lemon juice and greens like spinach or tomatoes. You can also toss in some herbs and a small amount of white tomato sauce. portion of fish

6 p.m., 6 p.m., 6 p.m Cooking Time: 15 minutes

Chapter 3

Egg Recipes

Breakfast Egg on Avocado

6 p.m., 6 p.m., 6 p.m Cooking Time: 15 minutes

Ingredients: 1 tsp garlic

powder 1/2 tsp sea salt

1/4 cup Parmesan cheese (grated or shredded) (grated or shredded) 1/4 tsp black pepper

3 medium avocados (cut in half, pitted, skin on) (cut in half, pitted, skin on) 6 medium eggs

Directions for Cooking:

Prepare biscuit tins and preheat the stove to 350oF.

To guarantee that the egg would fit inside the cavity of the avocado, gently scratch off 1/3 of the meat.

Place avocado on biscuit tin to guarantee that it faces with the top up.

Evenly season every avocado with pepper, salt, and garlic powder.

Add one egg on every avocado pit and embellishment tops with cheese.

Pop in the broiler and heat until the egg white is set, around 15 minutes.

Serve and enjoy.

Nutrition Information:

Calories per serving: 252; Protein: 14.0g; Carbs: 4.0g; Fat: 20.0g

Breakfast Egg-artichoke Casserole

Serves: 8 , Cooking Time: 35 minutes Ingredients: 16 large eggs

14 ounce can artichoke hearts, drained 10-ounce box frozen chopped spinach, thawed and drained well 1 cup shredded white cheddar

1 garlic clove,

minced 1 teaspoon salt

1/2 cup parmesan cheese 1/2 cup ricotta

cheese 1/2 teaspoon dried thyme

1/2 teaspoon crushed red pepper 1/4 cup milk

1/4 cup shaved onion

Directions for Cooking:

Lightly oil a 9x13-inch baking dish with cooking shower and preheat the broiler to 350oF.

In a huge blending bowl, add eggs and milk. Blend thoroughly.

With a paper towel, crush out the abundance dampness from the spinach leaves and add to the

bowl of eggs.

Into little pieces, break the artichoke hearts and separate the leaves. Add to the bowl of eggs.

Except for the ricotta cheddar, add remaining fixings in the bowl of eggs and blend thoroughly.

Pour egg combination into the arranged dish.

Evenly add dabs of ricotta cheddar on top of the eggs and afterward fly in the oven.

Bake until eggs are set and doesn't shake when shook, around 35 minutes.

Remove from the broiler and uniformly partition into proposed servings. Enjoy.

Nutrition Information:

Calories per serving: 302; Protein: 22.6g; Carbs: 10.8g; Fat: 18.7g

Brekky Egg-potato Hash

Serves: 2, Cooking Time: 25 minutes Ingredients: 1 zucchini, diced

1/2 cup chicken broth

½ pound cooked chicken 1 tablespoon olive oil 4 ounces shrimp

Salt and ground black pepper to taste 1 large sweet potato, diced 2 eggs

1/4 teaspoon cayenne pepper 2 teaspoons garlic powder 1 cup fresh spinach (optional) (optional)

Directions for Cooking: In a skillet, add the olive oil.

Fry the shrimp, cooked chicken and yam for 2 minutes.

Add the cayenne pepper, garlic powder and salt, and throw for 4 minutes.

Add the zucchini and throw for another 3 minutes.

Whisk the eggs in a bowl and add to the skillet.

Season utilizing salt and pepper. Cover with the lid.

Cook for 1 moment and add the chicken broth.

Cover and cook for an additional 8 minutes on high heat.

Add the spinach and throw for 2 additional minutes.

Serve immediately.

Nutrition Information:

Calories per serving: 190; Protein: 11.7g; Carbs: 2.9g; Fat: 12.3g

Dill and Tomato Frittata

Serves: 6, Cooking Time: 35 minutes Ingredients: Pepper and salt to

taste 1 tsp red pepper

flakes 2 garlic cloves, minced ½ cup crumbled goat cheese – optional 2 tbsp fresh chives, chopped 2 tbsp fresh dill,

chopped 4 tomatoes, diced 8 eggs, whisked 1 tsp coconut oil

Directions for Cooking:

Grease a 9-inch round baking dish and preheat broiler to 325oF.

In an enormous bowl, blend well all fixings and fill prepared pan.

Pop into the stove and heat until center is cooked through around 30-35 minutes.

Remove from stove and trimming with more chives and dill. Nutrition Information:

Calories per serving: 149; Protein: 13.26g; Carbs: 9.93g; Fat: 10.28g

Paleo Almond Banana Pancakes

Serves: 3, Cooking Time: 10 minutes Ingredients: ¼ cup almond flour ½ teaspoon ground cinnamon 3 eggs

1 banana, mashed

1 tablespoon almond butter 1 teaspoon vanilla

extract 1 teaspoon olive oil

Sliced banana to serve

Directions for Cooking: Whisk the eggs in a blending bowl until they become fluffy.

In another bowl, crush the banana utilizing a fork and add to the egg mixture.

Add the vanilla, almond spread, cinnamon and almond flour.

Mix into a smooth batter.

Heat the olive oil in a skillet.

Add one spoonful of the hitter and fry them on both sides.

Keep doing these means until you are finished with all the batter.

Add some cut banana on top before serving.

Nutrition Information:

Calories per serving: 306; Protein: 14.4g; Carbs: 3.6g; Fat: 26.0g

Chapter 3 Vegetable Recipes

Breakfast with Bananas and Coconuts serves 4 people and takes 3 minutes to prepare.

1 banana, ripe

1 cup desiccated coconut

coconut 1 quart of coconut milk

3 tablespoons chopped raisins 2 tblsp flax seed, ground 1 teaspoon vanilla extract a pinch of

a pinch of cinnamon

salt to taste nutmeg

Cooking Instructions: Combine all ingredients in a deep pan.

Allow for 3 minutes of simmering on low heat.

Place each item in its own container.

Put a label on it and put it in the fridge.

Allow to thaw at room temperature before microwaving to reheat.

Information about nutrition:

279 calories per serving; 25.46 grams of carbohydrates; 6.4 grams of protein; g of fat; 5.9 grams of fiber

Soup with basil and tomatoes

Cooking Time: 25 minutes, 2 servings

Season with salt and pepper to taste.

2 bay leaves, taste

12 cup unsweetened almond milk

12 tsp apple cider vinegar (raw) a third cup of basil leaves

a quarter cup of tomato paste

1 medium celery stalk, chopped 3 cups tomatoes

1 medium carrot, peeled and sliced

minced medium garlic clove

12 CUP ONION, WHITE

a tablespoon of vegetable broth

Cooking Instructions:

In a large saucepan, cook the vegetable stock over medium heat.

Cook for 3 minutes after adding the onions. Cook for another minute after adding the garlic.

Cook for 1 minute after adding the celery and carrots.

Add the tomatoes and bring the mixture to a boil. 15 minutes of simmering Combine the almond milk, basil, and straight leaves in a mixing bowl. To taste, season with salt and pepper.

Information about nutrition:

213 calories per serving; 42.0 grams of carbohydrates; 6.9 grams of protein; 3.9 grams of fat

Hummus with Butternut Squash

2 pounds butternut squash, seeded and halved Cooking Time: 15 minutes Ingredients: 2 pounds butternut squash, seeded and halved

1 tablespoon olive oil, peeled

a quarter cup of tahini lemon juice (two teaspoons) 2 garlic cloves, 2 garlic cloves, 2 garlic cloves, 2 garlic cloves

minced Season with salt and pepper to taste.

Cooking Instructions:

Preheat the broiler to 3000 degrees Fahrenheit.

Olive oil should be used to coat the butternut squash.

Place in a baking dish and bake in the oven for 15 minutes.

Place the cooked squash, along with the other ingredients, in a food processor.

Pulse until the mixture is completely smooth.

Place each item in its own container.

Make a note of it and keep it in the fridge.

Allow to come to room temperature before reheating in the microwave.

Serve with carrots or celery sticks as an accompaniment.

Information about nutrition:

115 calories per serving; 15.8 grams of carbohydrates; 2.5 grams of protein; 5.8 grams of fat; 6.7 grams of fiber

Jambalaya Cajun Soup serves 6 people and takes 6 hours to prepare.

14 cup Frank's spicy sauce

sauce a third of a teaspoon of Cajun seasoning

12 head cauliflower 2 cups okra 1 pound of hot Andouille sausages 2 bay leaves 4 oz. chopped chicken 1 lb. big raw and deveined shrimp

2 garlic cloves, diced

1 big can chopped organic tomatoes 4 peppers 1 big onion, diced

5 c. chicken broth

Cooking Instructions: Place the narrows leaves, very spicy sauce, Cajun preparation, chicken, garlic, onions, and peppers in a slow cooker.

Cook for 5 12 hours on low in a slow cooker.

After that, add the frankfurters and simmer for another 10 minutes.

Meanwhile, to create cauliflower rice, blitz the cauliflower in a food processor.

Fill the slow cooker halfway with cauliflower rice. Cooking time is 20 minutes.

Serve and have fun.

Information about nutrition:

155 calories per serving; 13.9 grams of carbohydrates; 17.4 grams of protein; 3.8 grams of fat

Chapter 4

Greek Style Collard Green Wrap

Cooking Time: 0 minutes, Serves: 4

12 block feta, cut into 4 (1-inch thick) strips for the wrap (4-oz)

12 cup diced purple onion

12 red bell peppers, medium

4 big collard green leaves, halved 1 medium cucumber, julienned 1 medium cucumber, julienned 4 large cherry tomatoes

8 whole kalamata olives, rinsed and halved

Ingredients for Tzatziki Sauce: 1 cup full-fat plain Greek yogurt

yogurt 1 tablespoon vinegar (white)

1 teaspoon powdered garlic

2 tablespoons olive oil 2 teaspoons minced fresh dill

cucumber, seeded and shredded (2.5 oz.)

entire) seasoning with salt and pepper to taste

Cooking Instructions:

Make the Tzatziki sauce first: after crushing the cucumber, try to squeeze out as much liquid as possible. Combine all sauce ingredients in a small dish and set aside to chill.

Prepare and chop all of the components for the wrap.

Spread one collard green leaf on a flat surface. 2 tbsp. Tzatziki sauce, spread in the middle of the leaf

14 of each of the tomatoes, feta, olives, onion, pepper, and cucumber should be layered. Place them on the leaf's main point, such as by stacking them high rather than spreading them out.

Fold the leaf in half like a tortilla. For the remaining components, repeat the procedure.

Serve and have fun.

Information about nutrition:

165.3 calories per serving; 7.0 grams of protein; 9.9 grams of carbohydrates; 11.2 grams of fat

Pizza with Portobello Mushrooms serves 4 people. Time to cook: 12 minutes

12 teaspoon red pepper flakes (optional)

a handful of basil leaves,

1 tblsp. black olives, diced

onion, medium,

1 green pepper, finely chopped

14 cup roasted yellow peppers, diced

12 cup shredded prepared nut cheese

cups gluten-free pizza sauce (made)

8 Portobello mushrooms, stems removed and cleaned

Cooking Instructions:

Preheat the toaster under the broiler.

Prepare a baking sheet by lightly oiling it. Remove from the equation.

Place 2 tablespoons of wrapped pizza sauce over the bottom of each Portobello mushroom cap, cap-side down. Add the nut cheddar and the other ingredients on top.

Broil for 12 minutes, or until wilted garnishes.

Information about nutrition:

578 calories per serving; 73.0 grams of carbohydrates; 24.4 grams of protein; 22.4 grams of fat

Roasted Root Veggies

Serves: 6, Cooking Time: 1 hour and 30 minutes

Ingredients: 2 tbsp olive oil

1 head garlic, cloves separated and peeled

1 large turnip, peeled and cut into ½-inch pieces

1 medium sized red onion, cut into ½-inch pieces

½ lbs. beets, trimmed but not peeled, scrubbed and cut into ½-inch pieces 1 ½ lbs. Yukon gold potatoes, unpeeled, cut into ½-inch pieces

½ lbs. butternut squash, peeled, seeded, cut into ½-inch pieces

Cooking Instructions: Combine all of the ingredients in a large mixing bowl and mix well

Grease 2 rimmed and enormous baking sheets. Preheat broiler to 425oF.

In an enormous bowl, blend all fixings thoroughly.

Into the two baking sheets, equitably partition the root vegetables, spread in one layer.

Season liberally with pepper and salt.

Pop into the stove and meal for 1 hour and 15 moment or until brilliant brown and tender.

Remove from broiler and let it cool for no less than 15 minutes before serving.

Information about the food:

Calories per Serving: 298; Carbs: 61.1g; Protein: 7.4g; Fat: 5.0g

Amazingly Good Parsley Tabbouleh\sServes: 4, Cooking Time: 15 minutes

Ingredients:

¼ cup chopped fresh mint

¼ cup lemon juice

¼ tsp salt

½ cup bulgur

½ tsp minced garlic 1 cup water

1 small cucumber, peeled, seeded and\sdiced 2 cups finely chopped flat-leaf parsley 2 tbsp extra virgin olive\soil 2 tomatoes, diced 4 scallions, thinly sliced Pepper to taste

Cooking Instructions: Combine all of the ingredients in a large mixing bowl and mix well

Cook bulgur as per bundle directions. Channel and put away to cool for no less than 15 minutes.

In a little bowl, blend pepper, salt, garlic, oil, and lemon juice.

Transfer bulgur into an enormous plate of mixed greens bowl and blend in scallions, cucumber, tomatoes, mint, and parsley.

Pour in dressing and throw well to coat.

Place bowl in ref until chilled before serving.

Information about the food:

Calories per Serving: 134.8; Carbs: 13g; Protein: 7.2g; Fat: 6g

Appetizing Mushroom Lasagna

Serves: 8, Cooking Time: 75 minutes\sIngredients:\s½ cup grated Parmigiano-Reggiano\scheese No boil lasagna noodles Cooking spray

¼ cup all-purpose flour

3 cups reduced fat milk, divided 2 tbsp chopped fresh chives, divided 1/3 cup less fat cream cheese

½ cup white wine

6 garlic cloves, minced and

divided 1 ½ tbsp. Chopped fresh thyme

½ tsp freshly ground black pepper, divided 1 tsp salt, divided

1 package 4 oz pre-sliced exotic mushroom

blend 1 package 8oz pre-sliced cremini mushrooms

1 ¼ cups chopped

shallots 2 tbsp olive oil, divided

1 tbsp butter

1 oz dried porcini

mushrooms 1 cup boiling water

Cooking Instructions: Combine all of the ingredients in a large mixing bowl and mix well

For 30 minutes, lower porcini in 1 cup extremely hot water. With a strainer, strain mushroom and hold liquid.

Over medium high fire, soften margarine on a fry skillet. Blend in 2 tbsp oil and for three minutes fry shallots. Add ¼ tsp pepper, ½ tsp salt, extraordinary mushrooms and cremini, cook for six minutes. Mix in 3 garlic cloves and thyme, cook briefly. Heat to the point of boiling as you pour wine by expanding fire to high and cook until fluid dissipates around a moment. Switch off fire and mix in porcini mushrooms, 1 tbsp chives and cream cheddar. Blend well.

On medium high fire, place a different medium estimated skillet with 1 tbsp oil. Sauté for a large portion of brief 3 garlic cloves. Then, at that point, heat to the point of boiling as you pour 2\s¾ cups milk and saved porcini fluid. Season with remaining pepper and salt. In a different bowl, whisk together flour and ¼ cup milk and fill skillet. Mix continually and cook until combination thickens.

In a lubed rectangular glass dish, pour and spread ½ cup of sauce, top with lasagna, top with half of mushroom blend and one more layer of lasagna. Rehash the layering system and on second thought of lasagna layer, end with the mushroom combination and cover with cheese.

For 45 minutes, heat the lasagna in a preheated 350oF stove. Decorate with chives before serving.

Information about the food:

Calories per Serving: 268; Carbs: 29.6g; Protein: 10.2g; Fat: 12.6g

Artichokes, Olives & Tuna Pasta\sServes: 4, Cooking Time: 15 minutes

Ingredients:\s¼ cup chopped fresh basil

¼ cup chopped green olives

¼ tsp freshly ground pepper

½ cup white wine

½ tsp salt, divided\s10-oz package frozen artichoke hearts, thawed and squeezed dry 2 cups grape tomatoes, halved

tbsp lemon juice

2 tsp chopped fresh rosemary 2 tsp freshly grated lemon zest 3 cloves garlic, minced 4 tbsp extra virgin olive oil,

divided 6-oz whole wheat penne pasta

8-oz tuna steak, cut into 3 pieces

Cooking Instructions: Combine all of the ingredients in a large mixing bowl and mix well

Cook penne pasta as indicated by bundle directions. Channel and set aside.

Preheat barbecue to medium high.

In bowl, throw and blend ¼ tsp pepper, ¼ tsp salt, 1 tsp rosemary, lemon zing, 1 tbsp oil and fish pieces.

Grill fish for 3 minutes for every side. Permit to cool and chip into scaled down pieces.

On medium fire, place a huge nonstick pan and hotness 3 tbsp oil.

Sauté remaining rosemary, garlic olives, and artichoke hearts for 4 minutes

Add wine and tomatoes, heat to the point of boiling and cook for 3 minutes while mixing once in a while.

Add staying salt, lemon juice, fish pieces and pasta. Cook until warmed through.

To serve, embellish with basil and enjoy.

Information about the food:

Calories per Serving: 127.6; Carbs: 13g; Protein: 7.2g; Fat: 5.2g
Serves: 4, Cooking Time: 35 minutes

Chapter 4 Pasta, Rice and Grains Recipes

Bell Peppers 'n Tomato-Chickpea Rice

Serves: 4, Cooking Time: 35 minutes

Ingredients:

2 tablespoons olive oil

1/2 chopped red bell pepper 1/2 chopped green bell pepper
1/2 chopped yellow

pepper 1/2 chopped red pepper

onions, medium

chopped 1 clove garlic, minced

cups cooked jasmine

rice 1 teaspoon tomato paste

1 cup

chickpeas salt to taste

1/2 teaspoon paprika

1 small tomato,

chopped Parsley for garnish

Cooking Instructions: Combine all of the ingredients in a large mixing bowl and mix well

In a huge blending bowl, whisk well olive oil, garlic, tomato glue, and paprika. Season with salt generously.

Mix in rice and prepare well to cover in the dressing.

Add remaining fixings and prepare well to mix.

Let salad rest to permit flavors to blend for 15 minutes.

Toss once again and change salt to taste if needed.

Garnish with parsley and serve.

Information about the food:

Calories per serving: 490; Carbs: 93.0g; Protein: 10.0g; Fat: 8.0g

Seafood and Veggie Pasta\sServes: 4, Cooking Time: 20 minutes

Ingredients:

¼ tsp pepper

¼ tsp salt

1 lb raw shelled shrimp 1 lemon, cut into wedges 1 tbsp butter

tbsp olive oil

5-oz cans chopped clams, drained (reserve 2 tbsp clam juice) (reserve 2 tbsp clam juice) 2 tbsp dry white wine

4 cloves garlic, minced\s4 cups zucchini, spiraled (use a veggie spiralizer) (use a veggie spiralizer) 4 tbsp Parmesan Cheese Chopped fresh parsley to garnish

Cooking Instructions: Combine all of the ingredients in a large mixing bowl and mix well

Ready the zucchini and spiralize with a veggie spiralizer. Organize 1 cup of zucchini noodle per bowl. Absolute of 4 bowls.

On medium fire, place a huge nonstick pan and hotness oil and butter.

For a moment, sauté garlic. Add shrimp and cook for 3 minutes until murky or cooked.

Add white wine, held shellfish squeeze and mollusks. Bring to a stew and keep stewing for 2 minutes or until half of fluid has vanished. Mix constantly.

Season with pepper and salt. Also if necessary add more to taste.

Remove from fire and equitably convey fish sauce to 4 bowls.

Top with a tablespoonful of Parmesan cheddar per bowl, serve and enjoy. Information about the food:

Calories per Serving: 324.9; Carbs: 12g; Protein: 43.8g; Fat: 11.3g

Breakfast Salad From Grains and Fruits

Serves: 6 , Cooking Time: 20 minutes Ingredients: ¼ tsp salt

¾ cup bulgur

¾ cup quick cooking brown rice 1 8-oz low fat vanilla yogurt 1 cup raisins

1 Granny Smith

apple 1 orange 1 Red delicious apple 3 cups water

Directions for Cooking: On high fire, place a huge pot and carry water to a boil.

Add bulgur and rice. Lower fire to a stew and cook for ten minutes while covered.

Turn off fire, put away for 2 minutes while covered.

In baking sheet, move and equitably spread grains to cool.

Meanwhile, strip oranges and cut into areas. Slash and center apples.

Once grains are cool, move to an enormous serving bowl alongside fruits.

Add yogurt and blend well to coat.

Enjoy your meal!

Information about the food:

Calories per Serving: 48.6; Carbs: 23.9g; Protein: 3.7g; Fat: 1.1g

Puttanesca Style Bucatini Serves: 4, Cooking Time: 40 minutes
Ingredients:

1 tbsp capers, rinsed tsp coarsely chopped fresh oregano 1 tsp finely chopped garlic 1/8 tsp salt

12-oz bucatini pasta cups coarsely chopped canned no-salt-added whole peeled tomatoes with their juice 3 tbsp extra virgin olive oil,

divided 4 anchovy fillets, chopped

8 black Kalamata olives, pitted and sliced into slivers

Cooking Instructions: Combine all of the ingredients in a large mixing bowl and mix well

Cook bucatini pasta as indicated by bundle headings. Channel, keep warm, and set aside.

On medium fire, place a huge nonstick pan and hotness 2 tbsp oil.

Sauté anchovies until it starts to disintegrate.

Add garlic and sauté for 15 seconds.

Add tomatoes, sauté for 15 to 20 minutes or until presently not watery. Season with 1/8 tsp salt.

Add oregano, tricks, and olives.

Add pasta, sautéing until warmed through.

To serve, sprinkle pasta with staying olive oil and enjoy. Information about the food:

Calories per Serving: 207.4; Carbs: 31g; Protein: 5.1g; Fat: 7g

Cinnamon Quinoa Bars

Serves: 4, Cooking Time: 30 minutes Ingredients: 2 ½ cups cooked

quinoa 4 large eggs

1/3 cup unsweetened almond milk 1/3 cup pure maple syrup

Seeds from ½ whole vanilla bean pod or 1 tbsp vanilla extract 1 ½ tbsp cinnamon

1/4 tsp salt

Cooking Instructions: Combine all of the ingredients in a large mixing bowl and mix well

Preheat stove to 375oF.

Combine all fixings into huge bowl and blend well.

In an 8 x 8 Baking skillet, cover with material paper.

Pour hitter equally into baking dish.

Bake for 25-30 minutes or until it has set. It ought not squirm when you softly shake the dish on the grounds that the eggs are completely cooked.

Remove as fast as conceivable from skillet and material paper onto cooling rack.

Cut into 4 pieces.

Enjoy all alone, with a little spread of almond or nut margarine or delay until it cools to partake in the following morning.

Information about the food:

Calories per serving: 285; Carbs: 46.2g; Protein: 8.5g; Fat: 7.4g

Creamy Alfredo Fettuccine

Serves: 4, Cooking Time: 25 minutes

Ingredients: Grated parmesan cheese

½ cup freshly grated parmesan

cheese 1/8 tsp freshly ground black pepper

½ tsp salt

1 cup whipping cream 2 tbsp butter

8 oz dried fettuccine, cooked and drained

Directions for Cooking: On medium high fire, place a major fry container and hotness butter.

Add pepper, salt and cream and tenderly bubble for three to five minutes.

Once thickened, switch off fire and right away mix in ½ cup of parmesan cheddar. Throw in pasta, blend well.

Top with one more cluster of parmesan cheddar and serve. Information about the food:

Calories per Serving: 202; Carbs: 21.1g; Protein: 7.9g; Fat: 10.2g

Greek Couscous Salad and Herbed Lamb Chops

Serves: 4, Cooking Time: 30 minutes

Ingredients: ¼ tsp salt

½ cup crumbled feta

½ cup whole wheat couscous 1 cup water

1 medium cucumber, peeled and

chopped 1 tbsp finely chopped fresh parsley

tbsp minced garlic

½ lbs. lamb loin chops, trimmed of fat 2 medium tomatoes, chopped 2 tbsp finely chopped fresh dill 2 tsp extra virgin olive oil 3 tbsp lemon juice

Cooking Instructions: Combine all of the ingredients in a large mixing bowl and mix well

On medium pan, add water and bring to a boil.

In a little bowl, blend salt, parsley, and garlic. Rub onto sheep chops.

On medium high fire, place a huge nonstick pan and hotness oil.

Pan fry sheep hacks for 5 minutes for each side or to wanted doneness. Once done, switch off fire and keep warm. On pot of bubbling water, add couscous. When bubbling, lower fire to a stew, cover and cook for two minutes.

After two minutes, switch off fire, cover and let it represent 5 minutes.

Fluff couscous with a fork and spot into a medium bowl.

Add dill, lemon juice, feta, cucumber, and tomatoes in bowl of couscous and throw well to combine.

Serve sheep cleaves with a side of couscous and enjoy.

Information about the food:

Calories per Serving: 524.1; Carbs: 12.3g; Protein: 61.8g; Fat: 25.3g

Chapter 5

Spanish Rice Casserole with Cheesy Beef

Serves: 2, Cooking Time: 32 minutes

Ingredients: 2 tablespoons chopped green bell

pepper 1/4 teaspoon Worcestershire sauce

1/4 teaspoon ground cumin 1/4 cup shredded Cheddar

cheese 1/4 cup finely chopped onion

1/4 cup chile sauce

1/3 cup uncooked long grain rice 1/2-pound lean ground beef 1/2 teaspoon salt 1/2 teaspoon brown sugar 1/2 pinch ground black pepper 1/2 cup water

1/2 (14.5 ounce) can canned tomatoes 1 tablespoon chopped fresh cilantro

Cooking Instructions: Combine all of the ingredients in a large mixing bowl and mix well

Place a nonstick pot on medium fire and earthy colored hamburger for

10 minutes while disintegrating meat. Dispose of fat.

Stir in pepper, Worcestershire sauce, cumin, earthy colored sugar, salt, chile sauce, rice, water, tomatoes, green ringer pepper, and onion.

Blend well and cook for 10 minutes until mixed and a piece tender. 3) Transfer to an ovenproof goulash and press down solidly. Sprinkle cheddar on top and cook for 7 minutes at 400oF preheated stove. Sear for 3 minutes until top is delicately browned.

4) Serve and appreciate with hacked cilantro.

Information about the food:

Calories per serving: 460; Carbohydrates: 35.8g; Protein: 37.8g; Fat: 17.9g

Tasty Lasagna Rolls

Serves: 6, Cooking Time: 20 minutes Ingredients: ¼ tsp crushed red pepper

¼ tsp salt

½ cup shredded mozzarella cheese

½ cups parmesan cheese,

shredded 1 14-oz package tofu, cubed

1 25-oz can of low-sodium marinara sauce 1 tbsp extra virgin olive oil 12 whole wheat lasagna noodles 2 tbsp Kalamata olives, chopped 3 cloves minced garlic 3 cups spinach, chopped

Cooking Instructions: Combine all of the ingredients in a large mixing bowl and mix well

Put sufficient water on a huge pot and cook the lasagna noodles as indicated by bundle guidelines. Channel, wash and put away until prepared to use.

In a huge skillet, sauté garlic over medium hotness for 20 seconds. Add the tofu and spinach and cook until the spinach shrivels. Move this blend in a bowl and add parmesan olives, salt, red pepper and 2/3 cup of the marinara sauce.

In a dish, spread a cup of marinara sauce on the base. To make the rolls, put noodle on a surface and spread ¼ cup of the tofu filling. Roll up and put it on the skillet with the marinara

sauce. Carry on in this manner until all of the lasagna noodles have been rolled.

Bring the stew to a boil in the container over high heat. Reduce the heat to medium and cook for an additional three minutes. Allow two minutes for the mozzarella to soften before adding the cheddar. Serve immediately.

Food-related information:

304 calories per serving; 39.2 grams of carbohydrates; 23 grams of protein; 19.2 grams of fat

Salad with Tortellini and Broccoli

12 servings Time to prepare: 20 minutes

Ingredients:

1 chopped red onion

1 cup sunflower seeds, finely chopped

1 pound of raisins

3 broccoli florets, trimmed from 3 heads 2 teaspoons apple cider vinegar

12 cup granulated sugar

a quarter-cup of mayonnaise

Tortellini with fresh cheese filling, 20 ounces

Cooking Instructions: In a large mixing basin, combine all of the ingredients and stir thoroughly.

Cook tortellini according to package instructions in a large saucepan of boiling water. Set aside after channeling and flushing with cold water.

To prepare your mixed greens dressing, whisk together the vinegar, sugar, and mayonnaise.

Combine red onion, sunflower seeds, raisins, tortellini, and broccoli in a large mixing dish. Toss in the dressing and toss to coat.

Take pleasure in your food!

Food-related information:

272 calories per serving; 38.7 grams of carbohydrates; 5.0 grams of protein; 8.1 grams of fat

Anti-Pasto Penne is a simple pasta dish.

4 servings 15-minute cooking time

Ingredients:

12 cup grated Parmigiano-Reggiano cheese, divided 14 cup pine nuts, toasted 8 oz. cooked and drained penne pasta

1 jar artichoke hearts, drained, cut, marinated, and quartered
1 jar sun-dried tomato halves packed in oil, drained and chopped 3 ounces prosciutto, diced

a third cup of pesto

12 cup Kalamata olives, pitted and chopped 1 red bell pepper, medium

Instructions for Cooking: In a large mixing basin, combine all of the ingredients and stir thoroughly.

Remove the films, seeds, and stem from the ringer pepper before slicing it. Place ringer pepper halves on a thwarted coated baking sheet, press someplace near hand, and sear for eight minutes in the oven. Remove the chicken from the broiler and place it in a fixed pack for 5 minutes before stripping and cutting.

In a mixing dish, combine the sliced chile pepper, artichokes, tomatoes, prosciutto, pesto, and olives.

In a large mixing bowl, combine 14 cup cheddar cheese and the pasta. Transfer to a serving plate and top with 14 cup cheddar cheese and pine nuts. Serve and have fun!

Food-related information:

606 calories per serving; 70.3 grams of carbohydrates; 27.2 grams of protein; 27.6 grams of fat

Porridge made with red quinoa and peaches

Cooking Time: 30 minutes Servings: 1 14 cup old fashioned rolled oats

14 cup quinoa (red)

12 gallon milk

12 cup of water

peeled and sliced peaches

Cooking Instructions: Place the peaches and quinoa in a small pan. Cook for 5 minutes after adding the water.

Time limit: 30 minutes

Cook until the oats are soft, then add the cereal and milk last. 3) Stir occasionally to prevent the porridge from sticking to the pan.

the pan's lowest portion

Information about nutrition: 456.6 calories per serving; 77.3 grams of carbohydrates; 16.6 grams of protein; and 9 grams of fat Servings: 2 Time to cook: 8 minutes

Recipes for Breads, Flatbreads, and Pizzas (Chapter 5)

Mixture of avocado with turkey Panini serves 2 people and takes 8 minutes to prepare.

Ingredients:

14 pound thinly sliced mesquite smoked turkey breast 2 red peppers, roasted and split into strips 1 cup fresh spinach leaves (distributed) 2 provolone cheese slices 2 ciabatta buns, 1 tablespoon olive oil

a quarter cup of mayonnaise

12 avocados, ripe

Cooking Instructions: In a mixing bowl, thoroughly combine mayonnaise and avocado.

Preheat the Panini press after that.

Slice the bread rolls into equal half and brush the insides of the bread with olive oil. Fill it with the following ingredients, piling them as you go: provolone, turkey breast, roasted red pepper, spinach leaves, avocado mixture, and the second bread slice.

Place the sandwich in the Panini press and grill for 5 to 8 minutes, or until the cheese has melted and the bread is crisp and ridged.

Food-related information:

546 calories per serving; 31.9 grams of carbohydrates; 27.8 grams of protein; 34.8 grams of fat

Servings: 1 Time to prepare: 20 minutes

12 slices of a medium cucumber, sliced lengthwise

12 ripe mangoes

salad dressing (tbsp)

choice 1 tortilla wrap made from whole wheat

2 tbsp oil for frying 1 inch thick piece of chicken breast roughly 6-inch in length

1 tbsp whole wheat flour

2–4 lettuce leaves, floured

season with salt and pepper to taste

Cooking Instructions: Cut a chicken breast into 1-inch strips and cook an aggregate of 6-inch strips. That would be the equivalent of two chicken pieces. Store

Chicken will be kept for future use.

Season the chicken with salt and pepper. Toss with a handful of whole wheat flour.

Place a small nonstick fry pan with hotness oil on medium heat. When the oil is heated, add the chicken fingers and fry until golden brown on both sides, about 5 minutes each side.

Place tortilla envelops in the broiler for 3 to 5 minutes while the chicken is cooking. Then remove it from the burner and place it on a platter.

Cut the cucumber in half lengthwise, using just 12 of it, and storing the rest. Remove the material from the cucumber, which has been split into quarters. Place the two cucumber slices on the tortilla wrap 1 inch from the edge.

Half of the mango should be sliced and the other half should be stored with the seeds. Remove the seeds from the mango and cut it into strips before placing it on top of the cucumber on the tortilla wrap.

Once the chicken is done, arrange it in a line with the cucumber.

Add a cucumber leaf and a salad dressing of your choosing.

Serve the tortilla wrap and take a bite.

Food-related information:

434 calories per serving; 10 grams of fat; 21 grams of protein; 65 grams of carbohydrates

6 servings 15-minute cooking time

Ingredients:

2 pita bread loaves

1 tbsp Olive Oil Extra Virgin 1/2 teaspoon sumac, with a little more for later seasoning with salt and pepper

1 Romaine lettuce heart

1 English cucumber, finely chopped

5 Roma tomatoes, chopped 5 green onions (white and green sections), chopped 5 radishes, thinly sliced 2 cups parsley leaves, chopped (stems removed) 1 cup fresh mint leaves, cut

Ingredients for the dressing:

1/3 cup Extra Virgin Olive Oil, juice of 1 1/2 limes seasoning with salt and pepper

1 tsp sumac powder

Quinoa Cinnamon Bars

Cooking Time: 30 minutes, Serves: 4 2 12 cup cooked peas, peas, peas, peas, peas, pe

quinoa a dozen big eggs

1/3 cup almond milk, unsweetened 1/3 cup maple syrup, undiluted

1 12 tbsp cinnamon 12 entire vanilla bean pod seeds or 1 tbsp vanilla extract

a quarter teaspoon of salt

Instructions for Cooking: In a large mixing basin, combine all of the ingredients and stir thoroughly.

Preheat the oven to 375 degrees Fahrenheit.

In a large mixing basin, combine all of the ingredients and mix well.

Cover an 8 × 8 baking pan with parchment paper.

In a baking dish, evenly distribute the batter.

Bake for 25-30 minutes, or until the cheese has hardened. When you gently shake the dish, it should not wiggle since the eggs are fully cooked.

Remove as soon as possible from the skillet and place on a cooling rack lined with parchment paper.

Cut each piece into four pieces.

Enjoy it on its own, with a little almond or nut margarine poured on top, or wait until the next morning to eat it.

Food-related information:

285 calories per serving; 46.2 grams of carbohydrates; 8.5 grams of protein; 7.4 grams of fat

Fettuccine Alfredo Creamy

Cooking Time: 25 minutes, Serves: 4

Grated parmesan cheese is one of the ingredients.

12 cup parmesan cheese, grated

1/8 teaspoon black pepper, freshly ground

12 teaspoon salt

1 quart of whipped cream 2 tablespoons butter

8 oz cooked and drained dry fettuccine

Cooking Instructions: Place a large fry container and heated butter on a medium high temperature.

Add the pepper, salt, and cream, and cook for three to five minutes, stirring occasionally.

Switch off the heat after the sauce has thickened and immediately stir in 12 cup of parmesan cheese. Toss in the noodles and well combine.

Serve with a final cluster of parmesan cheddar on top. Food-related information:

202 calories per serving; 21.1 grams of carbohydrates; 7.9 grams of protein; 10.2 grams of fat

Herbed Lamb Chops with Greek Couscous Salad

4 servings Time to prepare: 30 minutes

14 tsp salt, 14 tsp thyme, 14 tsp thyme, 14

12 cup feta cheese, crumbled

12 cup couscous (wholegrain) 1 quart of liquid

1 medium peeled cucumber

1 tablespoon fresh parsley, freshly chopped

1 tblsp garlic (minced)

12 pound trimmed fat lamb loin chops 2 tbsp fresh dill, coarsely chopped 2 medium tomatoes, chopped 2 tblsp olive oil (extra virgin) lemon juice, 3 tblsp

Directions for Cooking In a large mixing basin, thoroughly combine all of the ingredients.

Bring water to a boil in a medium sauce pan.

Salt, parsley, and garlic are combined in a small bowl. Rub the lamb chops with this mixture.

Place a large nonstick pan and plenty of heated oil on a medium high temperature.

Sheep chops should be pan fried for 5 minutes each side or until desired doneness is reached. When you're finished, turn off the heat and stay toasty. Add couscous to a saucepan of simmering water. Reduce the heat to a simmer, cover, and cook for two minutes after the mixture has started to bubble.

Switch off the fire after two minutes, cover it, and wait five minutes.

Fill a medium bowl halfway with couscous and fluff with a fork.

In a couscous bowl, toss together the dill, lemon juice, feta, cucumber, and tomatoes.

Serve with couscous and sheep cleaves.

Food specific information:

524.1 calories per serving; 12.3 grams of carbohydrate; 61.8 grams of protein; and 25.3 grams of fat

With Cheesy Beef in a Spanish Rice Casserole

2 people, 32 minutes to cook

2 tablespoons green bell peppers, chopped

pepper Worcestershire sauce, 1/4 teaspoon

1 tablespoon cumin powder shredded Cheddar cheese, 1/4 cup

onion, coarsely chopped 1/4 cup cheese

chile sauce (1/4 cup)

1/2 pound lean ground beef 1/3 cup long grain rice, uncooked 1 tsp. salt, 1 tsp. brown sugar black pepper, ground water (1/2 cup)

14.5 oz. canned tomatoes fresh cilantro, chopped

Directions for Cooking In a large mixing basin, thoroughly combine all of the ingredients.

Put an earthy colored hamburger in a nonstick saucepan on medium heat.

While the meat is dissolving, set aside 10 minutes. Fat should be removed.

Add the pepper, Worcestershire sauce, cumin, earthy colored sugar, salt, chile sauce, rice, water, tomatoes, green ringer pepper, and onion, and stir to combine.

Cook for 10 minutes, stirring occasionally, until fully combined and a piece is soft. 3) Press down firmly in an ovenproof goulash. Cook for 7 minutes at 400°F on a preheated burner with cheddar cheese on top. 3 minutes on the stovetop until the top is lightly browned.

4) Garnish with chopped cilantro before serving.

Food specific information:

460 calories per serving; 35.8 grams of carbs; 37.8 grams of protein; 17.9 grams of fat

Rolls of delicious Lasagna

6 portions 20 minutes of cooking time 14 teaspoon red pepper, crushed

salt (14 tsp)

12 cup mozzarella cheese (shredded)

12 cup grated parmesan

shredded 1 box cubed 14-ounce tofu

1 low-sodium marinara sauce can (25 ounces) 1 tablespoon olive oil (extra virgin) 12 lasagna noodle (whole wheat) 2 tblsp.

chopped Kalamata olives 3 garlic cloves, chopped 3 quarts chopped spinach

Cooking Instructions: Combine all of the ingredients in a large mixing bowl and mix well

Put sufficient water on a huge pot and cook the lasagna noodles as indicated by bundle guidelines. Channel, wash and put away until prepared to use.

In a huge skillet, sauté garlic over medium hotness for 20 seconds. Add the tofu and spinach and cook until the spinach shrivels. Move this blend in a bowl and add parmesan olives, salt, red pepper and 2/3 cup of the marinara sauce.

In a dish, spread a cup of marinara sauce on the base. To make the rolls, put noodle on a surface and spread ¼ cup of the tofu filling. Roll up and put it on the skillet with the marinara

sauce. Repeat until all of the lasagna noodles have been rolled.

Bring the stew to a boil in the pot over high heat. Reduce the heat to medium and continue cooking for three minutes more. Allow two minutes for the cheese to soften after being sprinkled with mozzarella. Warm it up and serve.

Food specific information:

304 calories per serving, 39.2 grams of carbohydrates, 23 grams of protein, and 19.2 grams of fat

Broccoli and Tortellini Salad

(12 people) 20 minutes of cooking time

Ingredients:

a chopped red onion

sunflower seeds, finely chopped 1 cup

a pound of raisins

3 broccoli florets (cut from 3 heads) 2 tbsp vinegar (apple cider)

12 cup sugar (white)

mayonnaise (12 cup)

Tortellini filled with fresh cheese, 20 oz.

Instructions for Cooking: In a large mixing bowl, combine all of the ingredients and mix thoroughly.

Cook tortellini according to manufacturer's instructions in a large pot of boiling water. Set aside after flushing the channel with cold water.

To make your mixed greens dressing, combine the vinegar, sugar, and mayonnaise.

Red onion, sunflower seeds, raisins, tortellini, and broccoli should all be mixed together in a large mixing bowl. Toss in the dressing to coat.

Have fun eating!

Food specific information:

272 calories per serving; 38.7 grams of carbohydrate; 5.0 grams of protein; and 8.1 grams of fat

Anti-Pasto Penne

4 portions 15 minutes of preparation time

Ingredients:

12 cup Parmigiano-Reggiano grated cheese, divided 14 cup pine nuts, toasted cooked and drained 8 oz. penne pasta

1 jar artichoke hearts (6 oz) drained, sliced, marinated, and quartered 1 jar sun-dried tomato halves in oil, drained and chopped 3 oz prosciutto (chopped)

pesto, 1/3 cup

12 c. Kalamata olives, pitted and chopped red bell pepper, medium

Directions for Cooking In a large mixing basin, thoroughly combine all of the ingredients.

Remove the films, seeds, and stem from the ringer pepper. Place ringer pepper parts on a foil-lined baking sheet, push somewhere close to hand, and sear for eight minutes in the oven. Remove from broiler and set aside for 5 minutes in a fixed pack before stripping and chopping.

In a mixing bowl, combine artichokes, tomatoes, prosciutto, pesto, and olives with the cleaved chile pepper.

14 cup cheddar cheese and pasta should be tossed together. Add 14 cup cheddar and pine nuts to a serving dish. Enjoy your meal!

Food specific information:

606 calories per serving; 70.3 grams of carbohydrate; 27.2 grams of protein; and 27.6 grams of fat

Peach Porridge with Red Quinoa

1 person, 30 minutes to prepare 14 cup rolled oats (old fashion)

14 c. quinoa (red)

milk, 12 cup

12 c.

peeling and slicing peaches

Place the peaches and quinoa in a small pan. Cook for another 10 minutes after adding water.

30-minute time limit

Cook until the oats are tender before adding the cereal and milk. 3) Stir the porridge occasionally to avoid it sticking to the pan.

the pan's lower section

Information about the food: 456.6 calories per serving; 77.3 grams of carbohydrate; 16.6 grams of protein; 9 grams of fat 2 people 8-Minute Preparation

Chapter 6

Bread, Flatbread, and Pizza Recipes

Turkey and Avocado Salad Panini serves two people and takes about eight minutes to prepare.

Ingredients:

14 lb. thinly sliced mesquite smoked turkey breast 2 red peppers, roasted and cut into strips 1 cup spinach leaves, whole and divided Provolone cheese, cut into two slices 2 ciabatta rolls, 1 tablespoon olive oil, divided

mayonnaise (1/4 cup)

12 avocados that have reached their full ripeness

Cooking Instructions: Combine mayonnaise and avocado in a bowl and crush completely.

The Panini press should then be preheated.

Spread olive oil on the insides of the bread rolls and slice them into equal parts. Then layer provolone, turkey breast, roasted red pepper, spinach leaves, and avocado mixture before covering with the other bread slice.

Place the sandwich in the Panini press and grill for 5 to 8 minutes, or until the cheddar has melted and the bread has become crisp and ridged.

Food specific information:

546 calories per serving; 31.9 grams of carbohydrate; 27.8 grams of protein; and 34.8 grams of fat

1 portion 20 minutes of cooking time

12 medium cucumber slices, cut lengthwise

12 mangoes, ripe

dressing for salad (tbsp)

choice 1 wrap made from whole wheat

2 tbsp oil for frying 1-inch thick chicken breast slice, about 6-inch in length

whole wheat flour (tbsp)

2–4 lettuce leaves dusted with flour

salt and pepper to taste

Cooking Instructions: Cut a chicken breast into 1-inch strips and cook 6 strips at a time. That's the equivalent of two chicken portions. Store

For future use, keep the chicken.

Pepper and salt the chicken. Incorporate whole wheat flour into your recipe.

Place a nonstick fry skillet and hotness oil on a medium fire. When the oil is hot, add the chicken fingers and fry for about 5 minutes on each side until golden brown.

Cook tortilla envelops for 3 to 5 minutes under the broiler while the chicken is cooking. Remove from the stove and place on a plate at that point.

Cut the cucumber lengthwise, using only 12 percent of it, and storing the rest. Remove the substance by slicing the cucumber into quarters. Place the cucumber slices 1 inch from the edge of the tortilla wrap.

Half of the mango should be sliced and the remaining half should be kept whole. Remove the seeds from the mango and slice it into strips before placing it on top of the cucumber on the tortilla wrap.

Place the chicken in a line with the cucumber once it's done cooking.

Sprinkle with salad dressing of choice, then add cucumber leaf.

Serve and enjoy your tortilla wrap.

Food specific information:

434 calories per serving; 10 grams of fat; 21 grams of protein; 65 grams of carbs

6 portions 15 minutes of preparation time

Ingredients:

Pita bread, 2 loaves

1 tblsp Olive Oil (Extra Virgin) 1 tsp sumac, plus a little extra for later seasonings

1 Romaine lettuce heart, 1 Romaine heart, 1 Romaine heart, 1 Romaine heart,

1 English cucumber, chopped 1 English cucumber

5 Roma tomatoes, chopped 5 green onions, chopped (both white and green parts) 5 radishes, stems removed, thinly sliced 2 CUP FRESH PARSLEY LEAVES, CRUMBLED (SEEDS REMOVED) 1 c. mint leaves, chopped

Ingredients for the sauce:

1/3 cup extra virgin olive oil, juice of 1 1/2 limes seasonings

1 tblsp. sumac powder

1/4 tsp ground cinnamon

scant 1/4 tsp ground allspice

Directions for Cooking:

For 5 minutes toast the pita bread in the toaster. And afterward fellowship into pieces.

In an enormous dish on medium fire, heat 3 tbsp of olive oil in for 3 minutes. Add pita bread and fry until cooked, around 4 minutes while throwing around.

Add salt, pepper and 1/2 tsp of sumac. Eliminate the pita chips from the hotness and put on paper towels to drain.

Toss well the cleaved lettuce, cucumber, tomatoes, green onions, cut radish, mint leaves and parsley in an enormous plate of mixed greens bowl.

To make the lime vinaigrette, whisk together all fixings in a little bowl.

Drizzle over salad and prepare well to cover. Blend in the pita bread.

Serve and enjoy.

Information about the food:

Calories per Serving: 192; Carbs: 16.1g; Protein: 3.9g; Fats: 13.8g

Garlic & Tomato Gluten Free Focaccia

Serves: 8, Cooking Time: 20 minutes

Ingredients:\s1 egg

½ tsp lemon

juice 1 tbsp honey

4 tbsp olive oil

A pinch of sugar

1 ¼ cup warm water\stbsp active dry yeast 2 tsp rosemary,

chopped 2 tsp thyme, chopped\stsp basil, chopped 2 cloves garlic,

minced 1 ¼ tsp sea salt

2 tsp xanthan gum

½ cup millet flour\scup potato starch, not flour 1 cup sorghum flour

Gluten free cornmeal for dusting

Directions for Cooking:

For 5 minutes, turn on the stove and afterward switch it off, while keeping broiler entryway closed.

In a little bowl, blend warm water and spot of sugar. Add yeast and whirl delicately. Leave for 7 minutes.

In an enormous blending bowl, whisk well spices, garlic, salt, thickener, starch, and flours.

Once yeast is finished sealing, fill bowl of flours. Speed in egg, lemon juice, honey, and olive oil.

Mix completely and place in a very much lubed square dish, cleaned with cornmeal.

Top with new garlic, more spices, and cut tomatoes.

Place in the warmed stove and let it ascend for a large portion of an hour.

Turn on broiler to 375oF and in the wake of preheating time it for 20 minutes. Focaccia is done once best are gently browned.

Remove from broiler and dish right away and let it cool.

Best served when warm.

Information about the food:

Calories per Serving: 251; Carbs: 38.4g; Protein: 5.4g; Fat: 9.0g Serves: 4, Cooking Time: 10 minutes

Ingredients:

Bibb lettuce,

halved 4 slices red onion

4 slices tomato

4 whole wheat buns, toasted 2 tbsp olive oil

¼ tsp cayenne pepper,

optional 1 garlic clove, minced

1 tbsp sugar

½ cup water

1/3 cup balsamic vinegar

4 large Portobello mushroom caps, around 5-inches in diameter

Directions for Cooking: Remove comes from mushrooms and clean with a sodden fabric.

Move into a baking dish with gill-side up.

In a bowl, blend completely olive oil, cayenne pepper, garlic, sugar, water and vinegar. Pour over mushrooms and marinate mushrooms in the ref for at minimum an hour.

Once the one hour is almost up, preheat barbecue to medium high fire and oil barbecue grate.

Grill mushrooms for five minutes for each side or until delicate. Treat mushrooms with marinade so it doesn't dry up.

To collect, put ½ of bread bun on a plate, top with a cut of onion, mushroom, tomato and one lettuce leaf. Cover with the other top portion of the bun. Rehash process with outstanding fixings, serve and enjoy.

Information about the food:

Calories per Serving: 244.1; Carbs: 32g; Protein: 8.1g; Fat: 9.3g

Serves: 4 , Cooking Time: 25 minutes

Ingredients:

1 bulb garlic

1 red bell pepper, halved and seeded 1 tbsp chopped fresh basil 1 tbsp olive oil tsp black pepper eggplants, sliced lengthwise 2 rounds of

flatbread or pita Juice of 1 lemon

Directions for Cooking:

Grease barbecue grind with cooking splash and preheat barbecue to medium high.

Slice highest points of garlic bulb and enclose by foil. Place in the cooler piece of the barbecue and dish for somewhere around 20 minutes.

Place chime pepper and eggplant cuts on the most sweltering piece of grill.

Grill for something like a few minutes each side.

Once bulbs are done, strip off skins of simmered garlic and spot stripped garlic into food processor.

Add olive oil, pepper, basil, lemon juice, barbecued red ringer pepper and barbecued eggplant.

Puree until smooth and move into a bowl.

Grill bread no less than 30 seconds for every side to warm.

Serve bread with the pureed plunge and enjoy.

Information about the food:

Calories per Serving: 213.6; Carbs: 36.3g; Protein: 6.3g; Fat: 4.8g Serves: 8, Cooking Time: 20 minutes

Ingredients:

½ tsp apple cider vinegar 3 tbsp olive oil 2 eggs

1 tsp baking powder 1 tsp salt 2 tsp xanthan gum ½ cup tapioca starch

¼ cup brown teff flour

¼ cup flax meal

¼ cup amaranth flour

¼ cup sorghum flour

¾ cup brown rice flour

Directions for Cooking:

Mix well water and honey in a little bowl and add yeast. Leave it for precisely 10 minutes.

In a huge bowl, blend the accompanying in with an oar blender: baking powder, salt, thickener, flax supper, sorghum flour, teff flour, custard starch, amaranth flour, and earthy colored rice flour.

In a medium bowl, whisk well vinegar, olive oil, and eggs.

Into bowl of dry fixings pour in vinegar and yeast combination and blend well.

Grease a 12-biscuit tin with cooking shower. Move mixture uniformly into 12 biscuit tins and pass on it for an hour to rise.

Then preheat stove to 375oF and prepare supper rolls until tops are brilliant brown, around 20 minutes.

Remove supper rolls from broiler and biscuit tins right away and let it cool.

Best served when warm.

Information about the food:

Calories per Serving: 207; Carbs: 28.4g; Protein: 4.6g; Fat: 8.3g

Serves: 4 , 30 Minutes of Preparation

Ingredients: 1 cup uncooked

quinoa 2 large eggs

½ medium onion,

diced 1 cup diced bell pepper

1 cup shredded mozzarella cheese 1 tbsp dried basil 1 tbsp dried oregano 2 tsp garlic powder 1/8 tsp salt

1 tsp crushed red peppers

½ cup roasted red pepper,

chopped* Pizza Sauce, about 1-2 cups

Directions for Cooking:

Preheat stove to 350oF.

Cook quinoa as per directions.

Combine all fixings (with the exception of sauce) into bowl. Blend all fixings well.

Scoop quinoa pizza combination into biscuit tin equally. Makes 12 muffins.

Bake for 30 minutes until biscuits become brilliant in shading and the edges are getting crispy.

Top with 1 or 2 tbsp pizza sauce and enjoy!

Information about the food:

Calories per Serving: 303; Carbs: 41.3g; Protein: 21.0g; Fat: 6.1g Serves: 8, Cooking Time: 45 minutes

Ingredients:

½ cup chopped walnuts

4 tbsp fresh, chopped rosemary 1 1/3 cups lukewarm carbonated water 1 tbsp honey ½ cup extra virgin olive

oil 1 tsp apple cider vinegar

3 eggs

5 tsp instant dry yeast granules 1 tsp salt

1 tbsp xanthan gum

¼ cup buttermilk

powder 1 cup white rice flour

1 cup tapioca starch

1 cup arrowroot starch

1 ¼ cups allpurpose Bob's Red Mill gluten-free flour mix

Directions for Cooking:

In an enormous blending bowl, whisk well eggs. Add 1 cup warm water, honey, olive oil, and vinegar.

While beating persistently, add the other fixings aside from rosemary and walnuts.

Continue beating. In the event that mixture is excessively solid, add a touch of warm water. Batter ought to be shaggy and thick.

Then add rosemary and pecans keep manipulating until equitably distributed.

Cover bowl of mixture with a perfect towel, place in a warm spot, and let it ascend for 30 minutes.

Fifteen minutes into rising time, preheat broiler to 400oF.

Generously oil with olive oil a 2-quart Dutch stove and preheat inside broiler without the lid.

Once batter is finished rising, eliminate pot from stove, and spot dough inside. With a wet

spatula, spread top of mixture uniformly in pot.

Brush highest points of bread with 2 tbsp of olive oil, cover Dutch broiler and heat for 35 to 45 minutes.

Once bread is done, eliminate from stove. What's more delicately eliminate bread from pot.

Allow bread to cool something like ten minutes before slicing.

Serve and enjoy.

Information about the food:

Calories per Serving: 424; Carbs: 56.8g; Protein: 7.0g; Fat: 19.0g

Tasty Crabby Panini

Serves: 4 , Cooking Time: 10 minutes

Ingredients: 1 tbsp Olive oil

French bread split and sliced diagonally

1 lb. blue crab meat or shrimp or spiny lobster or stone crab

½ cup celery ¼ cup green onion chopped 1 tsp Worcestershire sauce 1 tsp lemon juice 1 tbsp Dijon mustard

½ cup light mayonnaise

Directions for Cooking: In a medium bowl blend the accompanying completely: celery, onion, Worcestershire, lemon juice, mustard and mayonnaise. Season with pepper and salt. Then, at that point, tenderly include the almonds and crabs.

Spread olive oil on cut sides of bread and smear with crab blend prior to covering with another bread slice.

Grill sandwich in a Panini press until bread is crisped and ridged.

Information about the food:

Calories per Serving: 248; Carbs: 12.0g; Protein: 24.5g; Fat: 10.9g 6 portions Cooking Time: 0 minutes

Chapter 6 Salad Recipes

Balela Salad From the Middle East

6 portions Cooking Time: 0 minutes

Salad Ingredients:

1 jalapeno, finely chopped (optional)

1/2 green bell pepper, cored and chopped 2 1/2 cups grape tomatoes, slice in halves 1/2 cup sun-dried tomatoes

1/2 cup freshly chopped parsley leaves 1/2 cup freshly chopped mint or basil leaves 1/3 cup pitted Kalamata olives 1/4 cup pitted green olives

3 1/2 cups cooked chickpeas, drained and rinsed

3 –5 green onions, both white and green parts, chopped

Ingredients for the sauce:

garlic clove,

minced 1 tsp ground

sumac 1/2 tsp Aleppo pepper

1/4 cup Early Harvest Greek extra virgin olive oil 1/4 to 1/2 tsp crushed red pepper (optional) 2 tbsp lemon juice

tbsp white wine vinegar

Salt and black pepper, a generous pinch to your taste

Directions for Cooking:

combine as one the plate of mixed greens fixings in an enormous plate of mixed greens bowl.

In a different more modest bowl or container, combine as one the dressing ingredients.

Drizzle the dressing over the plate of mixed greens and delicately throw to coat.

Set to the side for 30 minutes to permit the flavors to mix.

Serve and enjoy.

Information about the food:

Calories per Serving: 257; Carbs: 30.5g; Protein: 8.4g; Fats: 12.6g

1 portion Cooking Time: 10 minutes

Ingredients: 0.5 oz chopped

walnuts 1 handful baby arugula

1 Persian cucumber, sliced into circles about ½-inch thick 3 oz halloumi cheese

5 grape tomatoes, sliced in half balsamic vinegar

olive

oil salt

Directions for Cooking:

Into 1/3 cuts, cut the cheddar. For 3 to 5 minutes each side, barbecue the sorts of cheddar until you can see barbecue marks.

In a plate of mixed greens bowl, add arugula, cucumber, and tomatoes. Sprinkle with olive oil and balsamic vinegar. Season with salt and prepare well coat.

Sprinkle pecans and add barbecued halloumi.

Serve and enjoy.

Information about the food:

Calories per serving: 543; Protein: 21.0g; Carbs: 9.0g; Fat: 47.0g
Serves: 4, Cooking Time: 0 minutes

Ingredients: ¼ tsp sea salt

¼ tsp ground cinnamon

½ tsp ground turmeric

¾ tsp ground ginger

½ tbsp extra virgin olive oil

½ tbsp apple cider vinegar 2 tbsp chopped green

onion 1/3 cup coconut cream

½ cup carrots, shredded

1 small head of broccoli, chopped

Directions for Cooking:

In an enormous plate of mixed greens bowl, blend well salt, cinnamon, turmeric, ginger, olive oil, and vinegar.

Add remaining fixings, throwing admirably to coat.

Pop in the ref for no less than 30 to an hour prior serving.
Information about the food:

Calories per serving: 90.5; Protein: 1.3g; Carbs: 4g; Fat: 7.7g

Serves: 4 , 15 minutes of preparation time

Ingredients: ½ cup red wine vinegar

1 tablespoon olive oil (extra virgin)

1 tbsp finely chopped celery

tbsp finely chopped red

onion 16 large ripe black olives

garlic cloves

2 navel oranges, peeled and segmented

4 boneless, skinless chicken breasts, 4-oz each 4 garlic cloves, minced 8 cups leaf lettuce, washed and dried Cracked black pepper to taste

Directions for Cooking:

Prepare the dressing by blending pepper, celery, onion, olive oil, garlic and vinegar in a little bowl. Whisk well to combine.

Lightly oil grind and preheat barbecue to high.

Rub chicken with the garlic cloves and dispose of garlic.

Grill chicken for 5 minutes for every side or until cooked through.

Remove from barbecue and let it represent 5 minutes prior to cutting into ½-inch strips.

In 4 serving plates, equitably orchestrate two cups lettuce, ¼ of the cut oranges and 4 olives for each plate.

Top each plate with ¼ serving of barbecued chicken, equally sprinkle with dressing, serve and enjoy.

Information about the food:

Calories per serving: 259.8; Protein: 48.9g; Carbs: 12.9g; Fat: 1.4g Serves: 6, Cooking Time: 0 minutes

Ingredients:

salt (14 tsp)

½ cup chopped red onion cup diced seedless cucumber 1 medium red bell pepper, diced 1/3 cup extra virgin olive oil 1/3 cup fresh dill, chopped 1/3 cup lemon juice

15oz cans of lentils

7oz cans of salmon, drained and flaked 2 tsp Dijon mustard Pepper to taste Directions for Cooking:

In a bowl, combine as one, lemon juice, mustard, dill, salt and pepper.

Gradually add the oil, ringer pepper, onion, cucumber, salmon pieces and lentils.

Toss to cover evenly.

Information about the food:

Calories per serving: 349.1; Protein: 27.1g; Carbs: 35.2g; Fat: 11.1g Serves: 4 , Cook Time: 3 minutes

Ingredients:

0.10 lbs of toasted and chopped hazelnut

0.45 lb of trimmed green beans ¼ lb mozzarella, ripped into chunks 1 shallot, sliced thinly 1 tbsp fig jam or relish

tbsp balsamic vinegar

3 tbsp extra virgin olive oil 6 small figs, quartered

Small handful of basil leaves, torn

Directions for Cooking:

For a few minutes, whiten beans in salted water. Then, at that point, eliminate the water, wash with cold faucet water, channel and let dry on top of kitchen towel.

Once the beans are dried, put on a food platter and add basil, hazelnuts, mozzarella, shallots and figs.

To make dressing, utilize a medium lidded container and add your decision of preparing, olive oil, fig jam and vinegar. Cover the container and shake energetically prior to pouring over the salad.

Information about the food:

Calories per Serving: 294.8; Fat: 17.6g; Protein: 12.7g; Carbs: 21.4g Serves: 2 , Cook Time: 0 minutes Ingredients:

½ cup coarsely chopped pistachio

½ cup sweet potato, spiralized 1 red bell pepper, diced 1 red bell pepper, julienned 1 ripe fuyu persimmon, diced 1 tbsp chili powder 2 fuyu persimmon, sliced 3 tbsp lime juice

4 cups mixed greens a pinch of chipotle powder salt to taste

Directions for Cooking:

In a plate of mixed greens bowl, blend and organize persimmons, chime pepper and yams. Set aside.

In a food processor, puree salt, lime juice, chipotle powder, stew powder, diced persimmon and diced ringer pepper until smooth and creamy.

Pour over salad, prepare to mix.

Serve and enjoy.

Information about the food:

Calories per Serving: 467.4; Fat: 15.4g; Protein: 11.3g; Carbs: 70.9g 6 pcs. Cook Time: 0 minutes

Ingredients:

¼ cup chopped fresh

mint 1 2/3 cups boiling water

1 cucumber, peeled, seeded and chopped 1 cup bulgur

1 cup chopped fresh parsley 1 cup chopped green onions 1 tsp salt 1/3 cup lemon

juice 1/3 cup olive oil

3 tomatoes, chopped

Ground black pepper to taste

Directions for Cooking:

In a huge bowl, combine as one bubbling water and bulgur. Let douse and save for an hour while covered.

After 60 minutes, throw in cucumber, tomatoes, mint, parsley, onions, lemon squeeze and oil. Then, at that point, season with dark pepper and salt to taste. Throw well and refrigerate for one more hour while covered before serving.

Information about the food:

Calories per serving: 185.5; Fat: 13.1g; Protein: 4.1g; Carbs: 12.8g Serves: 4, Cooking Time: 10 minutes

Chapter 7 Beans Recipes

Bean and Toasted Pita Salad

4 portions Cooking Time: 10 minutes

Ingredients:

3 tbsp chopped fresh mint

3 tbsp chopped fresh parsley 1 cup crumbled feta

cheese 1 cup sliced romaine lettuce

½ cucumber, peeled and

sliced 1 cup diced plum tomatoes cups cooked pinto beans, well drained and slightly warmed Pepper to taste

tbsp extra virgin olive oil 2 tbsp ground toasted cumin seeds 2 tbsp fresh lemon juice 1/8 tsp salt 2 cloves garlic, peeled

2 6-inch whole wheat pita bread, cut or torn into bite-sized pieces

Directions for Cooking:

In huge baking sheet, spread torn pita bread and prepare in a preheated 400oF stove for 6 minutes.

With the rear of a blade, crush garlic and salt until glue like. Add into a medium bowl.

Whisk in ground cumin and lemon juice. In a consistent and slow stream, pour oil as you whisk persistently. Season with pepper.

In a huge serving of mixed greens bowl, blend cucumber, tomatoes and beans. Yet again pour in dressing, throw to cover well.

Add mint, parsley, feta, lettuce and toasted pita, throw to blend and serve.

Information about the food:

Calories per serving: 427; Protein: 17.7g; Carbs: 47.3g; Fat: 20.4g

Beans and Spinach Mediterranean Salad

Serves: 4, Cooking Time: 30 minutes Ingredients:

1 can (14 ounces) water-packed artichoke hearts, rinsed, drained and quartered

can (14-1/2 ounces) no-salt-added diced tomatoes, undrained 1 can (15 ounces) cannellini beans, rinsed and drained 1 small onion, chopped 1 tablespoon olive oil 1/4 teaspoon

pepper 1/4 teaspoon salt

1/8 teaspoon crushed red pepper flakes 2 garlic cloves, minced tablespoons Worcestershire sauce 6 ounces fresh baby spinach (about 8 cups) Additional olive oil, optional

Directions for Cooking: Place a pot on medium high fire and hotness for a minute.

Add oil and hotness for 2 minutes. Mix in onion and sauté for 4 minutes. Add garlic and sauté for another minute.

Stir in flavors, Worcestershire sauce, and tomatoes. Cook for 5 minutes while blending ceaselessly until sauce is reduced.

Add the spinach, artichoke hearts, and beans and mix well. Sauté for 3 minutes, or until the spinach has wilted and the other ingredients are heated.

Serve and have fun.

Information about nutrition:

187 calories per serving; 8.0 grams of protein; 30.0 grams of carbohydrates; 4.0 grams of fat

Recipes for Seafood in Chapter 8

Grilled Calamari and Berries

4 servings, 5 minutes to prepare

14 cup dried cranberries (optional)

a quarter cup of extra virgin olive oil

14 cup extra virgin olive oil

14 cup almonds, sliced

12 oz. lemon juice

12 pound calamari tube, cleaned 34 cup blueberries 1 granny smith apple

1 tablespoon fresh lemon juice, thinly sliced

apple cider vinegar (tbsp.) 6 cups spinach, fresh to taste freshly grated pepper to taste with sea salt Cooking Instructions:

Blend the tablespoon of lemon juice, apple juice vinegar, and more virgin olive oil in a small basin to produce the vinaigrette. Season with salt and pepper to taste. Remove from the equation.

Turn the grill to medium heat and cook the meshes for a minute or two.

Combine the olive oil and calamari tube in a large mixing basin. Season the calamari with a generous amount of pepper and salt.

Place the prepped and oiled calamari on a preheated mesh grill pan and cook until the calamari is cooked or translucent. This will take around two minutes on each side.

While you wait for the calamari to cook, combine almonds, cranberries, blueberries, spinach, and the thinly sliced apple in a large dish of mixed greens. Toss into the mix.

Remove the cooked calamari from the grill and place it on a cutting board. Toss onto the plate of mixed greens bowl, cut into 14-inch thick rings.

Drizzle vinaigrette over salad and toss well to coat.

Serve and have fun!

Information about nutrition:

567 calories per serving; 24.5 grams of fat; 54.8 grams of protein; 30.6 grams of carbohydrates

Noodles with Cajun Garlic Shrimp 2 people in a bowl, 15 minutes to prepare Ingredients: 12 tsp

1 sliced onion, salted

1 red pepper, 1 red onion

1 tablespoon butter, sliced

1 garlic clove

1 teaspoon granules

powdered onion big zucchinis, sliced into noodle strips 1 teaspoon paprika 20 large shrimps, deveined and deshelled 3 garlic cloves, minced

a tsp of ghee

a smidgeon of cayenne

a sprinkling of red pepper flakes

Cooking Instructions:

Blend the onion powder, garlic granules, pepper chips, cayenne pepper, paprika, and salt together to make the Cajun seasoning. Toss in the shrimp to coat them with spice.

Heat the ghee in a pan and sauté the garlic. Continue to sauté for 4 minutes after adding the red pepper and onions.

Cook until the Cajun shrimp is misty. Remove from the equation.

Heat the spread in a separate container and sauté the zucchini noodles for three minutes.

Place the Cajun shrimp on top of the zucchini noodles to assemble.

Information about nutrition:

712 calories per serving; 30.0 grams of fat; 97.8 grams of protein; 20.2 grams of carbohydrates

Bacon-creamed fish Chowder

1 1/2 pound fish 1 1/2 pound cod 1 1/2 pound cod 1 1/2 pound cod 1 1/2 pound cod 1 1/2 pound cod 1 1/2 pound cod 1 1/2 pound cod 1 1/2 pound cod

1 1/2 teaspoon thyme, dry

1 big carrot, finely chopped 1 tbsp butter, sliced into tiny pieces 1 large onion, chopped 1 teaspoon salt, divided 1/2 cup peeled and diced baked potato 3 bacon slices (uncooked)

4 1/2 cups water 3/4 teaspoon freshly ground black pepper, divided

leaves of bay

4 cups reduced-fat milk (2% fat)

Cooking Instructions: Combine the water and inlet leaves in a large pan and simmer. Toss in the fish. Cover and continue to cook until the tissue chips easily with a fork. Remove the fish from the pan and chop it into large pieces. Remove the cooking liquid and set it aside.

Cook the bacon until it is crisp on a medium-hot Dutch burner. Remove the bacon and save the drippings. Set aside the bacon, which has been smashed. In a pan with the bacon drippings, combine the potato, onion, and carrot and simmer for 10 minutes over medium heat. Allow to boil while adding the cooking liquid, inlet leaves, 1/2 teaspoon salt, 1/4 teaspoon pepper, and thyme. Reduce the heat to low and simmer for 10 minutes. Stir in the milk and continue to cook until the potatoes are tender but not bubbling. Add the fish, 1/2 teaspoon of salt, and 1/2 teaspoon of pepper. Remove the leaves that are too thin.

Serve with the smashed bacon on top.

Information about nutrition:

400 calories per serving; 34.5 grams of carbohydrates; 20.8 grams of protein; 19.7 grams of fat

Halibut Pouches with Cucumber-Basil Salsa

Cook Time: 17 minutes (serves 4)

8 cups mustard greens, stems removed Ingredients: lime, finely cut into 8 pieces 2 tsp extra virgin olive oil

4–5 quartered and trimmed radishes 4 filets of skinless halibut, 4 ounce 4 big basil leaves, fresh

Optional: cayenne pepper to taste Season with salt and pepper to taste.

Ingredients for Salsa:

12 cup cucumber, diced

12 fresh basil leaves, freshly chopped 2 tsp lime juice, freshly squeezed Season with salt and pepper to taste.

Preheat the oven to 400 degrees Fahrenheit.

Make 4 parts of 15 x 12-inch square forms to use as material sheets. Overlap fifty-fifty and unroll pieces on the table the long way. 3) Season halibut filets with salt, pepper, and cayenne pepper, if using. 4) Place 12 cup mustard greens just to one side of the crease running longwise. Finish with a basil leaf on top of the mustard greens and a lime sliced. 14 radishes should be layered around the greens. Season with pepper and salt and drizzle with 12 tsp oil. A halibut fillet cut should be placed on top. 5) Fold the material paper over the filling and pleat the edges of the material paper from one end to the other end, as if making a calzone. Squeeze the wrinkled material paper to seal the finish. 6) Repeat the procedure with the remaining fixings until you have four pieces of material sheets stuffed with halibut and greens.

Place pockets in a baking dish and cook on the stove for 15 to 17 minutes, or until halibut is flaky.

While you wait for the halibut pockets to cook, create the salsa by combining all of the ingredients in a medium dish.

When the halibut is done, remove it from the broiler and create a rip in the top. Keep an eye out for the steam, which is quite hot. Similarly, divide the salsa and pour 14 tablespoons on top of the halibut through the incision you've made. 10) Finally, serve and enjoy.

Calories per serving: 335.4; protein: 20.2 g; fat: 16.3 g; carbohydrates: 22.1 g

White Sea Dill Relish Bass

4 servings, 12 minute cook time Ingredients: 12 tbsp chopped white onion

12 teaspoon fresh dill, chopped

1 quartered lemon

1 tsp Dijon mustard

1 tsp lemon juice mustard

1 teaspoon drained pickled baby capers

4 fillets of white sea bass, 4 oz.

Preheat the oven to 375 degrees Fahrenheit.

In a small bowl, combine the lemon juice, mustard, dill, escapades, and onions. 3) Cut four pieces of aluminum foil and place one filet on each foil. 4) For each fish, squeeze a lemon slice.

5) Divide the dill spread into four equal portions and sprinkle evenly over the fillet. 6) Carefully fold the foil over the fish and place it in the oven.

7) Bake for 10–12 minutes, or until fish is well done. 8) Transfer to a serving tray, remove the foil, and serve. Information about nutrition:

115 calories per serving; 7 grams of protein; 1 gram of fat; 12 grams of carbohydrates 4 servings Time to prepare: 20 minutes

Recipes for Poultry and Meat in Chapter 9

Chicken Soup for Vegetable Lovers

4 servings Time to prepare: 20 minutes

12 CUP BABY SPROUT INGREDIENTS: 12 CUP BABY SPROUT

a tablespoon of orzo (tiny pasta)

14 cup white wine, dry

12 tsp Italian spice 1 14 oz low sodium chicken broth 2 plum tomatoes, diced 1/8 tsp salt 1 shallot, 1 shallot, 1 shallot, 1 shallot

1 small onion, chopped

8 oz chicken tenders, diced zucchini

1 tbsp olive oil (extra virgin)

Cooking Instructions: 1) In a large saucepan, heat the oil over medium heat and add the chicken.

For 8 minutes, mix occasionally until seared. In a plate, move. Remove everything from the room. 2) In a similar saucepan, combine thee

zucchini, Italian flavoring, shallot and salt and

mix regularly until the vegetables are relaxed, around 4 minutes. 3) Add the tomatoes, wine, stock and orzo and increment the hotness to high to carry the combination to bubble. Decrease the hotness and

simmer.

4) Add the cooked chicken and mix in the spinach last. 5) Serve hot.

Nutrition Information:

Calories per Serving: 207; Carbs: 14.8g; Protein: 12.2g; Fat: 11.4g Servers: 10, Cook Time: 1 hour and 15 minutes

Ingredients:

½ cup red wine

1 ½ cups chicken stock or more if needed 1 cup olive oil

1 cup tomato sauce

pc, 4lbs whole chicken cut into pieces 1 pinch dried oregano or to taste 10 small shallots,

peeled 2 bay leaves

cloves garlic, finely

chopped 2 tbsp chopped fresh parsley

2 tsps butter

Salt and ground black pepper to taste

Directions for Cooking:

Bring to a heat up a huge pot of softly salted water. Blend in the shallots and let bubble uncovered until delicate for around three minutes. Then, at that point, channel the shallots and dunk in cool water until no longer warm.

In one more huge pot over medium fire, heat spread and olive oil until gurgling and softened. Then sauté in the chicken and shallots for 15 minutes or until chicken is cooked and shallots are soft and translucent. Then add the chopped garlic and cook for three mins more.

Then add narrows leaves, oregano, salt and pepper, parsley, pureed tomatoes and the red wine and let stew briefly prior to adding the chicken stock. Mix prior to covering and let cook for 50 minutes on medium-low fire or until chicken is tender.

Nutrition Information:

Calories per Serving: 644.8; Carbs: 8.2g; Protein: 62.1g; Fat: 40.4g Serves: 4, Cooking Time: 30 minutes

Ingredients:

Pepper and salt to taste

1 lb. ham, coarsely

chopped 24 oz frozen sweet peas 4 cup ham stock

¼ cup white wine 1 carrot, chopped

coarsely 1 onion,

chopped coarsely 2 tbsp butter, divided

Directions for Cooking:

On medium chimney a medium pot and hotness oil. Sauté for 6 minutes the onion or until delicate and translucent.

Add wine and cook for 4 minutes or until almost evaporated.

Add ham stock and bring to a stew and stew consistently while covered for 4 minutes.

Add peas and cook for 7 minutes or until tender.

Meanwhile, in a nonstick fry dish, cook to a seared fresh the ham in 1 tbsp margarine, around 6 minutes. Eliminate from fire and set aside.

When peas are delicate, move to a blender and puree. Get back to pot, keep cooking while at the same time preparing with pepper, salt and ½ of crisped ham. When soup is to your ideal taste, switch off fire.

Transfer to 4 serving bowls and embellishment uniformly with crisped ham.

Information about the food:

Calories per Serving: 403; Carbs: 32.5g; Protein: 37.3g; Fat: 12.5g 4 portions Cooking Time: 12 minutes

Ingredients:

¼ cup basil, finely shredded

14 cup extra virgin extra virgin extra virgin extra virgin extra virgin extra virgin extra virgin extra

½ cup mustard

¾ lb. fresh apricots, stone removed, and fruit diced 1 shallot, diced small

1 tsp ground cardamom 3 tbsp raspberry vinegar 4 pork chops Pepper and salt

CPSIA information can be obtained
at www.ICGtesting.com
Printed in the USA
BVHW010025070422
633551BV00016BB/869